" I see many of my patients within the pages of this book. Many are young women whose lives were forever changed when they were diagnosed with M.S. Many of them have shared stories of loss and uncertainty for the future yet they found the courage to pursue something new. Adaptive Yoga under the gentle guidance of Mindy Eisenberg has given them a NEW sense of SELF. I applaud her tireless commitment to this invaluable program and congratulate her on the publication of this much appreciated book. She has given her students something that they feared might be forever lost. "

MARGIE LEONARD, RN, MSCN, MIND CENTER, FARMINGTON HILLS, MICHIGAN

" A program of active exercise and often formal physical and occupational therapy are integral and important parts of a comprehensive and multidisciplinary approach to the care of patients with multiple sclerosis as well as many other chronic neurological diseases. A large number of my patients have been involved in various yoga programs and the benefits are clear. Yoga helps them physically, providing help with balance, core and extremity strength and with coordination. Perhaps of equal importance many report beneficial effects on their mood and outlook. In this book, Mindy Eisenberg provides guidelines on yoga which can be used as part of an active supervised program or a self-guided approach, that may prove helpful to patients as well, I am sure, to others who have no major neurological disorders but are looking for a program to benefit their general and mental health. "

—ROBERT P LISAK, MD, FRCP (E), FAAN, FANA, PARKER WEBBER CHAIR IN NEUROLOGY,
PROFESSOR OF NEUROLOGY, PROFESSOR OF IMMUNOLOGY AND MICROBIOLOGY,
WAYNE STATE UNIVERSITY SCHOOL OF MEDICINE, DETROIT, MI

" Mindy Eisenberg has been a role model for those teaching adaptive yoga. In addition, her energy and drive to provide free yoga to those living with multiple sclerosis has motivated hundreds of people to use yoga as a tool to better their lives. Her grace, compassion and years of service have inspired those souls stepping into the yoga path. Mindy's book *Adaptive Yoga Moves Any Body* is an easy to follow guide for anyone living with or without a physical limitation; a way to improve their mobility and have a brighter tomorrow. "

NATHALIE SLOANE, DEVELOPMENT DIRECTOR, MULTIPLE SCLEROSIS FOUNDATION

" Mindy's passion for making yoga accessible to individuals with different abilities is rooted deep in her compassion for others, enthusiasm and positive energy. Over the years, yoga with Mindy has helped me to develop better posture and core strength, improved body awareness and breathing techniques. "

ERICA COULSTON, PRESIDENT, WALK THE LINE TO SCI RECOVERY INC, C6/7 SCI SURVIVOR

" *Adaptive Yoga Moves Any Body* is a well written book that will be easy to use from the beginning yoga student to the more advanced devote. Mindy Eisenberg has taken Yoga and made it easy and fun with demonstrative photos and descriptions that make each yoga position easy to understand and duplicate. This book is very well suited for patients with Multiple Sclerosis as well as for many other neurological conditions. I would recommend this book to my patients and also to anyone else interested in beginning yoga or continuing their yoga journey. "

BHUPENDRA O. KHATRI, MD., MEDICAL DIRECTOR, THE REGIONAL MULTIPLE SCLEROSIS CENTER, MILWAUKEE, WI
AUTHOR OF THE AWARD WINNING BOOK, *HEALING THE SOUL.*

" *Adaptive Yoga Moves Every Body* offers yoga poses and sequences that are adapted to individual needs in a user friendly format, ranging from mat yoga to standing sequences with the wall, to chair, and to restorative poses. Whether your practice is chair yoga for the wheelchair or the office, this book shows you how to do it. Yoga is available to every body and yet not all yoga practices are suited to every body. *Adaptive Yoga Moves Every Body* by Mindy Eisenberg shows how yoga can be accessible to students of all ages and abilities. This book offers clear instruction and photos with a variety of models as well as easy to follow sequences. Written with humor and heart, *Adaptive Yoga Moves Every Body*, is a gem for yoga students and yoga teachers alike. "

KAREN O'DONNELL CLARKE, ERYT500, PYT1000, CERTIFIED KRIPALU YOGA
AND INTEGRATIVE YOGA THERAPIST

" Mindy Eisenberg's *Adaptive Yoga Moves Every Body* book is perfectly said. Mindy comes with Authenticity, compassion, and purpose. *Adaptive Yoga Moves Every Body* will make such a difference in all populations. Coming from an Emergency Responder population I can speak to her ability to calm the mind and body to allow for the inside-out healing to begin. It has been an honor to have Mindy come into my life and to see her ability to work through *Adaptive Yoga Moves Every Body*. I encourage everyone to use *Adaptive Yoga Moves Every Body* in all parts of their life. Thank You Mindy for all that you do. Sparkles, Love, & Kindness. "

MICHELLE E. REUGEBRINK, PROFESSIONAL INTEGRATIVE HEALTH COACH & MINDFULNESS
BASED STRESS REDUCTION TEACHER

Adaptive Yoga
Moves Any Body

Publisher: Orange Cat Press
Project Editor: Katherine Phillips
Cover and numerous additional photographs by Elayne Gross Photography
Additional Photographer: Lauren McRae
Designer: Eric Keller Design

Manufactured in the United States of America
Library of Congress Control Number: 2015942207
Eisenberg, Mindy.
       Adaptive yoga moves any body : created for people with MS
       and neuromuscular conditions a great introduction for all / Mindy Eisenberg:
       foreword by J. Matthew Voci, MD

ISBN: 978-0-692-43243-3

1. Adaptive Yoga. 2. Yoga Therapy. 3. Multiple Sclerosis. 4. Neuromuscular Conditions. 5. CAM.   I. Title.

Yoga Moves MS

Precautions: The yoga skills, techniques, and ideas in this book are not a substitute for medical care, or personal instruction from a qualified instructor. Please consult your physician before beginning your yoga practice, especially if you have a serious or chronic health care problem, abnormal blood pressure, a back injury, are pregnant, or have had surgery. The precautions listed are guidelines only. Any application of the contents of this book, including techniques and suggestions is at the reader's sole discretion and risk.

Adaptive Yoga
Moves Any Body

Mindy Eisenberg

Blessings for health and healing.
Mindy Eisenberg

ORANGE CAT PRESS

Dedicated to my beautiful mother

Linda Lee Weingarten

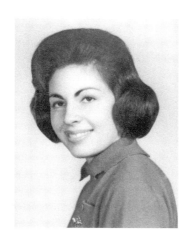

TABLE OF CONTENTS

ACKNOWLEDGEMENTS

With Gratitude

Gratitude is integral to living a rich, open-hearted life. Although my yogic path began over twenty-one years ago, teaching adaptive yoga for the last eleven years has been a life changing, exhilarating experience. For that, I am so grateful.

I am fortunate to be blessed with a team comprised of special individuals, colleagues, students, and professionals readily offering their talent, intellect, and love. Each one of them contributed to *Adaptive Yoga Moves Any Body.*

Since we met five years ago to brainstorm and flesh out the purpose of this book, my dear friend and colleague, Julie Levinson, has been by my side every step of the way. She lifted my energy when it was waning, and generously filled her free hours to brainstorming sessions. She prodded me to stay the course when I had my doubts or was overwhelmed with the task at hand. I never imagined myself as an author, but she intuitively knew this had to be done.

I have witnessed how yoga provides a healing path for my students. The thousands of sessions as their instructor have provided me with hope for the future that those with multiple sclerosis (MS) and neuromuscular conditions can live a quality life. My knowledge about adaptive yoga is the cumulative result of my teaching experience with my students and co-instructors. My students' presence and influence can be sensed on nearly every page of this book. Their participation is the primary reason why a wide spectrum of readers will benefit from

Acknowledgements

this book. Student photos and quotes clearly show their enthusiasm and demonstrate than "any body" can do yoga. I almost broke out in tears of happiness at the sight of my students cheering for each other as they patiently took turns modeling for the camera. A special thank you to those who gave their time and smiles to the photos including: Wanda Baum, Anne Bennett, Jodi BuWalda, Cynthia Cohen, Rene D'Ortenzio, Llindsay Dzngel, Jodi Ganley, Ed Gregory, Rebecca Guerra, Shirley Hardy, Rebecca Hernandez, Denise Hurtig, Peggy Johnson, Leslie Kaiser, Ina Katz, Lynn Kughn, Suzanne Kypros, Terri Kudwa, Suzanne Kypros, Lori Flowers, Kwana McBurrows, Carla McKeen, Dawn Monlleo, Mary Nunn, Carolyn Price, Tracey Robertson, Kathy Roe, Margo Rubens, Deborah Silverstein, Patricia Traczyk, Marcia Williams, Barbara Vandette, Glenna Wotherspoon, Linda Wdowiak, Lawrence Yaple, and Charles Zuccarini.

Yoga Moves MS (YMMS) is a non-profit community and movement that we started to help fundraise and support our adaptive yoga for MS classes. I cannot express enough gratitude to Dr. J. Matthew Voci, Chair and cheerleader for YMMS and our annual fundraiser. He has taken our grassroots movement to another level. His strategic planning and leadership, with his sincere passion for his patients and the neurological community, are a driving force behind the growth of adaptive yoga therapy. Please enjoy reading his preface to this book.

YMMS partners with the Multiple Sclerosis Foundation, a non-profit organization, to fund YMMS classes and ensure that they are available to those who could not otherwise afford yoga therapy. Without the support of Nathalie Sloane, Alan Segaloff, Alma Henry, and other MSF staff, our classes would not exist.

This book is a conglomeration of my years of practice and my learning from some of the most talented yoga instructors in the country. Matthew Sanford is one of my most important adaptive yoga instructors and inspired me with his strength to overcome great challenges, his powerful teaching style, and philosophy. Karen O' Donnell Clarke is one of the most adept yoga for MS instructors in this country. She dedicates herself to conducting national adaptive yoga teacher trainings, and I have been fortunate to be a part of them as a student and an assistant. I still find it useful to quote Eric Small, author of Yoga For MS, ten years after attending his trainings at the International Association of Yoga Therapists conference. Doug Keller, a nationally recognized expert yoga therapist, has taught me many yoga therapy concepts and techniques over several years of attending his trainings. Lynn Medow encouraged me to teach yoga for MS. I love her as a friend, teacher, colleague, and her work with the Yoga by Design Foundation. Numerous Karma Yoga studio kula instructors have shaped my yoga practice and career. Rabbi Rachel Lawson Shere is an important teacher on my spiritual path, and a great supporter of my work. I have quoted, sourced, or referenced material originating from publications and authors including: *Yoga for MS* by Dr. Lauren Fishman and Eric Small; *Mudras-Yoga in Your Hands* by Gertrud Hirschi; Jon Kabat Zinn's, *Full Catastrophe Living* and *Wherever You Go There You Are*; Yoga Therapy manuals by Doug Keller; *The Psoas Book* by Liz Koch; *Mudras for Healing and Transformation* by Joseph and Lilian Le Page; and *Waking: A Memoir of Trauma and Transcendence* by Matthew Sanford.

This book has had the gift of many pairs of eyes and minds. Joelle Shandler, gave me a kick start by introducing me to a meticulous editor, Maureen Dunphy who took me through the first round of edits. Over a year and half ago, Kate Phillips, a dedicated yoga practitioner and dear friend, enthusiastically stepped in to edit the next several revisions to completion with her gift of intellect, common sense, organization, detail, and perseverance. We had several fun yet intense, highly interactive sessions, practicing the poses as we edited the pose pages and sections in this book. In addition to his creative content, my designer, Eric Keller, has offered many thoughtful suggestions to enrich the experience for readers. Sara Davidson Flanders and Susann Spilkin, my knowledgeable and creative colleagues, contributed their gift of words and suggestions to the text. I am forever grateful to my

Acknowledgements

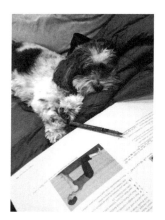

Yogi Garfield Eisenberg, Editor in Chief, hard at work

additional readers and contributors for their invaluable input including, Chris Briney, Marcy Fisher, Ernest Gifford, Lori Flowers, Terri Kudwa, Pat Lucas, Angela Mackensen, Michael Rice, Dr. James Voci, and Cindy Weingarten.

Several photographic sessions took place for this book at Rasa Yoga. I am indebted to Patricia Keros and Todd Tesen for their generosity of space. Lauren McRae, an adventurous student of photography accepted the challenge to capture images during the first of many photo sessions. Elayne Gross, who graciously volunteers her services at all of our YMMS fundraisers, contributed with her warmth and professional creative eyes, as she photographed the cover and multiplicity of photos in this book. Thank you to Village Yoga of Franklin for providing their studio for the videos that compliment this book. Jon Kopacz, the videographer, has dedicated much thought and time to their creation.

Finally, I thank my family, who exuded great patience while I crafted this book. My cousins, Joyce and Jeffrey, supplied the location for some of the videos and showed great understanding when I postponed lunch dates and outings. My in-laws, Nanny and Papa Eisenberg, in Arizona invited me to draft several sections of this book in their Scottsdale backyard. While Julia, my daughter, has been at college for much of the process, she sent her sweet messages of encouragement from afar, and tolerated and encouraged my work while she was home during summer breaks from college. Noah, my wise son, quietly put up with my hours working at the kitchen table and in front of the fireplace. While he claims his meals were scant during my writing and editing days, I choose to view this time as promoting his independence. Lastly and most importantly, I thank my husband of over 30 years, Scott, for his love, encouragement, and steady nature.

Garfield, my sweet furry buddy, who passed away on February 5, 2015, is *furever* missed. He spent many hours at my ankles or on book pages supporting my authorship of this book.

CHAPTER 1

Sharing the Beauty of Yoga

I am honored and excited to share the beauty of yoga with you. It has changed my life and the lives of so many others close to my heart. Whatever your reason for choosing this book, the practices herein will change your life. Instructing people who have multiple sclerosis (MS) and neuromuscular conditions has been one of the most rewarding gifts in my life. My students are my inspiration and I take great pride in our growing Yoga Moves community. They bring light to darkness, laughter to tears, strength to weakness, courage to fear, inspiration to despair, and healing to suffering. They make me feel as though I am the luckiest yoga instructor on the planet.

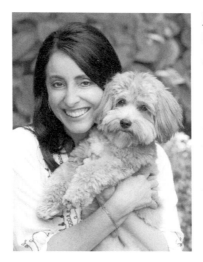

Although I have been practicing and studying yoga for over twenty-one years, my personal journey toward adaptive yoga began with my experiences as the daughter of a woman with severe physical challenges. My mother had a progressive form of MS, and was confined to a wheelchair for over 25 years. From my perspective, there were limited ways to increase her comfort and to maintain her strength and flexibility. I knew there had to be better options to improve her quality of life.

After completing my first teacher training, I was invited to volunteer as a yoga instructor for a support group of individuals with MS at a prominent neurological center. The participants took to yoga immediately and we formed a separate class for them as well as others interested in adaptive yoga. Although it was too late to help my mother, I quickly realized

Sharing the Beauty of Yoga

how the yoga classes immeasurably improved my students' sense of self-worth, capability, and well-being. They found that they moved more steadily, felt energized and serene, and they had a lot of fun. This epiphany carried me headlong into further studies to help this eager and underserved group. Thus, Yoga Moves MS was born. Since that first class, I have seen hundreds of my students with varying ranges of physical and cognitive abilities reap the rewards of the Yoga Moves program. I'd like you to enjoy the same benefits.

Why did I write this book? Very simply, my Yoga Moves students asked me to write a guide for them. They enjoyed how they felt during and after completing a class, and wanted to continue their practice at home. Experience showed them that the benefits of yoga dramatically increased with more frequent practice. They needed a way to remember

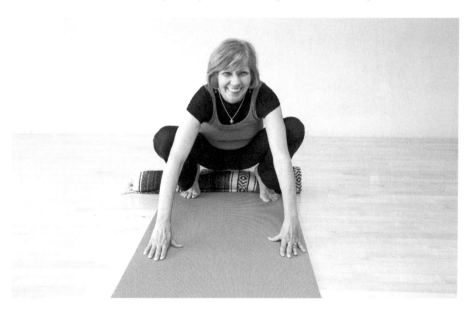

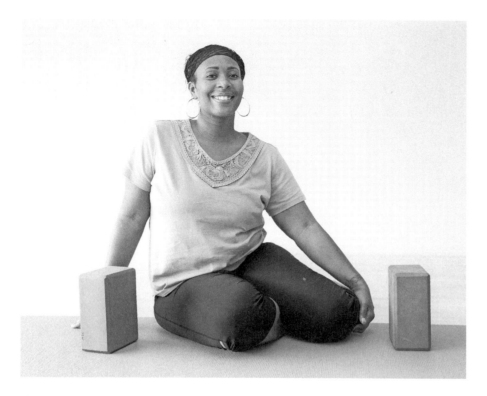

the poses and techniques and asked me for a few photos with accompanying instructions.

The more I spoke with other yoga instructors, practitioners, and medical professionals about the idea for an adaptive yogabook, the more it became apparent that there was a need for a comprehensive, user-friendly guide. With their simple request, my students unknowingly sent me on a five-year journey researching and writing *Adaptive Yoga Moves Any Body* to honor their appeal.

Who can benefit from this book? The principles of adaptive yoga can be applied to any body, and individuals with a variety of needs can benefit from a regular adaptive yoga practice. For example, the same symptoms my Yoga Moves students with MS experience are often manifested in others with various neuromuscular conditions. Rather than be defined by a condition or disease, Yoga Moves students feel more in touch with their humanity, and more comfortable with themselves. Most likely you will find yourself or someone you care

Sharing the Beauty of Yoga

about in this list of people who can benefit from *Adaptive Yoga Moves Any Body*:

- Any body with movement challenges
- Individuals seeking a gentle practice
- Individuals with MS, and a range of neuromuscular conditions
- Caregivers or family members of those with movement challenges
- Individuals new to yoga
- Experienced yogis who desire a home reference for adaptive yoga
- Yoga instructors seeking to learn how to adapt yoga for their students

The yoga classroom is a learning laboratory for both students and instructors. *Adaptive Yoga Moves Any Body* brings my knowledge together in one place, empowering you to tailor traditional postures to fit your unique needs and abilities. I have taught and studied adaptive yoga for over a decade. Rather than align with a particular yoga style, I apply lessons from different trainings, experiences, and settings to Yoga Moves classes, and observe what works best for my students and for you.

What is yoga? Yoga is the art and science of you. It nourishes your mind, strengthens your body, and elevates your spirit. The word "yoga"

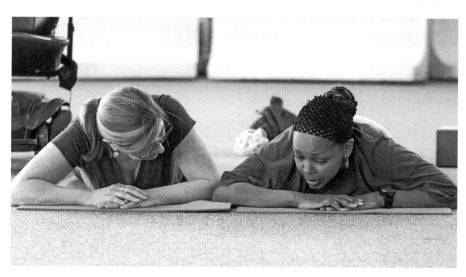

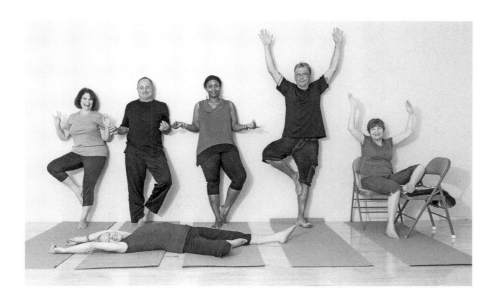

actually means "to join" in Sanskrit, as in to integrate, or form a
union between your mind, your body, and your spirit. Yoga connects
a physical practice (*asana*), breathing techniques (*pranayama*), and
meditation. It is not a religious belief system, and it can mean different
things to different people. Yogic philosophy traces its ancient roots
back 5000 years to what is now India. More recently, Western culture
has embraced yoga, with an emphasis on its physical poses. But it is
much more than just a workout routine. A conscious breathing practice
connects with mindful movement for a heightened sense of peace and
well-being. The more you become self-aware, the more readily you can
listen to what your body needs on any given day. Think of yourself as
a musician and your body as your instrument. Yoga will help you tune
that instrument so it plays harmoniously.

What is Adaptive Yoga? Since every body is unique, and each
individual's practice is different, essentially all yoga is adaptive to
some extent. However, those with movement challenges require a
more creative approach to traditional postures. With adaptive yoga,
a range of physical postures becomes accessible to a greater number
of practitioners.

In this book, traditional standing poses are presented with

Sharing the Beauty of Yoga

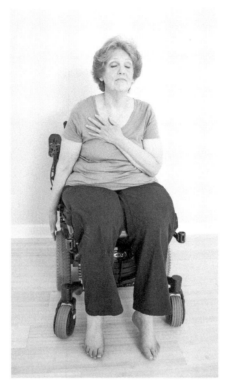

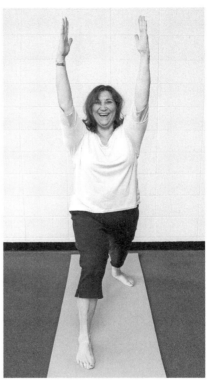

adaptations seated in a chair or lying down on a mat. Likewise, traditional seated poses that are commonly practiced on the mat are adapted so that individuals receive similar benefits when they are practiced in a chair. Props such as blankets, chairs, yoga straps, and blocks expand the accessibility of many fundamental yoga postures.

Adaptive yoga helps stability, comfort, and confidence in a pose. It doesn't push you beyond your physical limitations to achieve some unattainable idealized goal. Rather, it helps you believe in your own capabilities. With creativity and an open mind, yoga can be adapted to benefit any body. The possibilities are endless.

Why are people afraid of yoga? Ironically, people are afraid to try yoga, when actually, it often helps decrease anxiety and tension. Prospective students have said that they have held onto informational flyers about Yoga Moves classes for weeks, months, or even years before they take the plunge into their first class. Perhaps they are intimidated when they catch glimpses of bodies in twisty, curvy, mindboggling yoga poses.

A common misunderstanding is that flexibility is required before beginning a yoga practice. Actually, the reverse is true: flexibility is one of the many benefits of yoga, but it is not a requirement to embark on a practice.

Healing through yoga is not about fancy poses. Yoga is not "one size fits all." It fits all body types whether flexible or stiff, short or tall, muscular or lean, and able to ambulate with or without a cane, walker or wheelchair.

Why is yoga for you? Yoga enables you to help yourself, compliments your medical care, and gives you hope. With adaptive yoga, the many benefits of a seemingly impossible practice are within reach. As you begin the *Adaptive Yoga Moves Any Body* journey, you are offering yourself a pathway toward improved health and well-being.

Yoga can mitigate several physical symptoms of MS and neuromuscular conditions. The benefits individuals experience from yoga may include improved strength, flexibility, posture, balance, focus, speech, circulation, respiration, digestion, elimination, and pelvic floor health, along with decreased anxiety, tension, fatigue, numbness, spasticity, and other aches and pains. It can also provide overall coping skills to contend with these symptoms.

This is your time to take care of yourself. My students often state the greatest benefit of yoga is the private "me only" time carved out of their day and week. I can see the difference in how they feel when they use yoga to help themselves. Each one benefits in their own way, receiving what they need on a given day. Any student might leave class more peaceful, centered, or lively. Don't let your condition define you. Let yoga help you improve your health and quality of life.

CHAPTER 2

*Yoga has changed my life and my lifestyle. Before I start my day,
I have a routine of breathing, stretching, and meditation.*

MARCIA, YOGA MOVES STUDENT

How to Use This Book

Getting Started

I wish I could be in the room with you when you practice. After all, actions speak louder than words. However, in my absence, I hope this book and the related videos give you the tools you need to experience the difference yoga can make in your life, and enable you to say with conviction, "Yes, I can!"

All you need to bring to practice is an open mind, an open heart, self-love, and no judgment about what is good or bad, right or wrong.

Find a quiet space where you will not be interrupted, and perhaps, where you can conveniently store your props. Wear comfortable clothes. A fancy outfit is not required, but if it puts you in the mood to move, go for it. Ideally, begin at least two hours after your last meal,

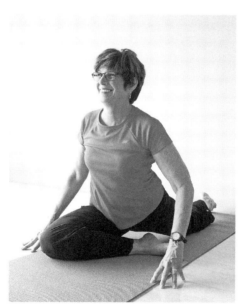

and empty your bladder before you start. Establish a routine with a regular time of day to practice. The more frequently you practice, the more benefits you will gain.

Ask yourself, "What does my mind and body need today?" Each day can be different. Take into account your schedule, how you slept and ate the previous day, and current stressors in your life, including any injuries or ailments. If you are feeling lethargic, a rejuvenating practice may be just what you need to enliven you. If you are getting over a recent cold, a more restorative practice may be appropriate. You will first need to decide if you are able to safely venture onto the yoga mat.

Transitional sequences to demonstrate how Yoga Moves students transfer down to the earth,

How to Use This Book

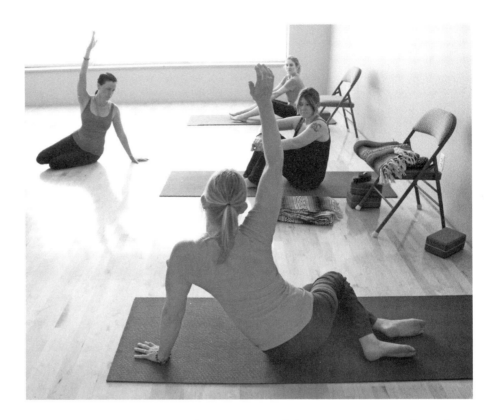

and return to the chair are found in "Playful, Empowering, and Healing Sequences."

BOOK ORGANIZATION

Each chapter focuses on key elements for a comprehensive yoga practice. My students and I demonstrate poses throughout this book. Think of us as your classmates and yoga buddies. Remember, each body will express a pose in its own unique way. You may not look exactly as the instructions describe, and you may not look exactly like the photos. In a photographic instructional book, it is tempting to only look at the photos. Resist the urge to practice a pose prior to reading the instructions. They contain valuable information for you to safely and effectively practice Yoga Moves.

Chapter 3 - Guiding Principles Yoga unifies mind, body, and spirit, and the book is organized to help you engage all three in your practice both on and off the mat. "Guiding Principles" informs you of the philosophy, wisdom, and ideas behind this unification. Before beginning your yoga journey, it is highly recommended and encouraged that you familiarize yourself with these concepts. They can be applied throughout your day, not just in your yoga practice.

Chapter 4 - Breath Practice A critical part of yoga practice is integrating your breath with the poses. It creates more space in your body for ease of movement. It helps you relax into a difficult posture. It invites a mindful and soulful practice.

Chapter 5 – Alignment for Life Alignment for Life describes postural and alignment fundamentals that are important to integrate with your daily movement patterns both as you are active and at rest. Optimal posture and alignment prevents injury and pain, and allows healthy energy to flow through your body.

Chapter 6 - Warm Up, Tune Up, Loosen Up Beginning the physical postures, "Warm Up, Tune Up, Loosen Up" provides necessary and simple ways to awaken your body. The warm-up sections are organized by body part from head to toe. These can either be integrated into your daily activities, used as a yoga practice by themselves, or can be performed before entering postures found in "Adaptive Poses."

Chapter 7 - Adaptive Poses An alphabetical listing of the yoga poses and their adaptations comprise the largest portion of this book. Some poses are energizing to build strength and stability, while restorative poses are relaxing and replenish energy. As you read "Adaptive Poses," know that you are not expected to remember the details, and can refer to them at any time.

Chapter 8 – Hand Gestures
These are simple yet powerful hand gestures that often are integrated at the beginning or ending of a yoga practice, or can be used at any

How to Use This Book

time outside your yoga practice. Also known as *mudras,* these can be very empowering and stimulate healing energetic qualities.

Chapter 9 - Playful, Empowering, and Healing Sequences

The sequences pull it all together for you by offering a variety of combinations, with themes, descriptions, and functions to help you choose among them. They are structured with options for poses and warm-ups in a chair, on a yoga mat, and standing. The videos on the website, *yogamovesms.org*, can help you with some of the sequences. You may wish to print a copy of your chosen sequence to cross-reference while watching a video.

YOGA MOVES CHAPTER FEATURES

Within each chapter you will find detailed descriptions of what you need to know for each entry.

Primary Benefits

For each pose, general benefits are listed to give you an idea how a pose helps others, and may benefit you. Taking into account that any and every body is different, you may experience more or varied benefits. During and after each pose, allow time to note how you feel.

Precautions

The listed precautions are general. They are not specific or exhaustive, but should be considered before practicing a pose. Always practice within your personal and physical limits. Take into account any recent injury or diagnosis as you formulate your own practice. If you are not comfortable with a pose, do not attempt it without the assistance of a qualified yoga instructor. Trust your intuition.

Before embarking on your yoga journey, discuss with your health care practitioner any breathing practice, warm-up, meditation, or pose that is in question, and show them photos and instructions to clarify what to avoid or modify.

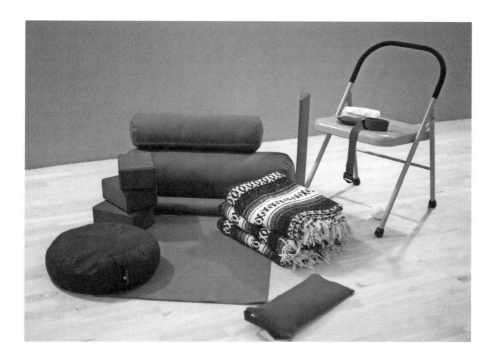

Props

Yoga poses can become more accessible with the use of props. They support, stretch, and provide a sense of direction and comfort, so that you can fully experience pose benefits and achieve an optimal state of physical alignment. Read the instructions and variations for each pose. Once you choose a pose adaptation, have the required props handy. You can often substitute with items you may have around your home. Commonly used props and their uses include:

- Meditation cushion to provide a comfortable seat while meditating, and to raise the hips above the knees
- Yoga mat to soften the ground, to delineate your practice area, and to provide stability
- Foam blocks to provide resistance, support, or to keep your hands closer to the earth
- Bolsters (or large pillows) to provide support and comfort
- Blankets to cushion knees, head, or buttocks
- Sand, rice, or bean bags in various sizes and weights to place over feet, palms, belly, and/or hips in restorative poses

How to Use This Book

- Yoga dumbbells to ease the load on your wrists
- Eye pillow or mask to improve relaxation while in restorative poses
- Washcloth (or hand towel) to provide cushioning for, or to wedge behind, a bent knee for comfort
- Yoga strap (or an old tie or bathrobe sash) to provide support for legs or shoulders, facilitate a stretch, or provide resistance in a posture
- Chair(s) or wheelchair to elevate the earth for seated postures, and to provide support during your practice *(Note: Poses may be practiced in a wheelchair. However, when possible, transfer to a chair to better support your posture.)*
- Tennis ball to massage feet or tight muscles
- Wall to provide support or resistance

Instructions

Read through each instruction thoroughly prior to practicing. The main steps are provided in numerical order. Refer to the steps at your own pace. Take time to melt into each pose and notice any sensations. With intention and attention, slowly move into and out of a pose. At times you will find that, with coordinated breath and mindful movement, your body will relax into a pose as you let go of tension. For many of the

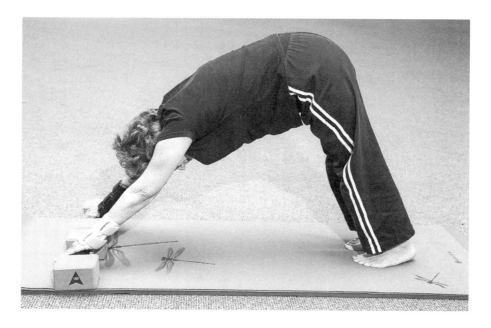

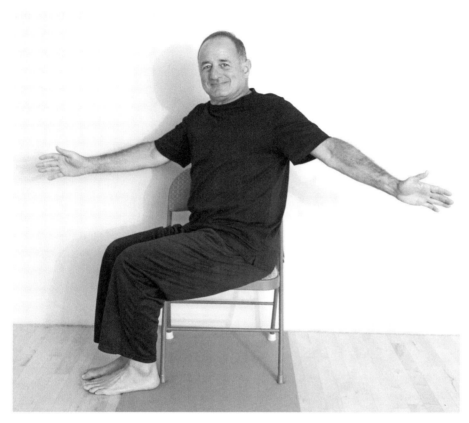

poses, the instructions state to enjoy a pose for 3 to 5 breaths. This is a guideline. Very simple poses can be more challenging by remaining in them for longer than the suggested time.

Instructions always begin on the right side of the body for asymmetrical poses. After practicing on the right side, repeat the pose instructions on the left side of your body.

Adaptations and Variations

These are provided to expand the accessibility of each breath, warm-up, pose, and mudra to fit your abilities. Examine the photos together with the descriptions and instructions to decide which option is best for you. The photos show the general shape of the pose, but do not illustrate all adaptations and variations. Take into account that every body is different. One variation is not necessarily any better than another, and each offers similar benefits to a traditional pose version.

How to Use This Book

You are nurturing yourself through your practice, not competing against your body's limitations. Over time you may create or design a new modification that suits your body even better. I encourage you to send me an email describing your creative modifications to *yogamovesms.org*. They may end up in the next edition.

To best evaluate which option to use first, read through the offerings. One might jump out to you as familiar or desirable. If not, try the one whose directions make the most sense to you. Trust your instincts, listen to your body, and be open to possibilities.

As with the poses, the instructions for adaptations and variations state to practice on the right side of the body for asymmetrical poses. To maintain balance, make sure to practice the adaptation on the left side as well.

Videos

Go to yogamovesms.org for videos that complement this book.

CHAPTER 3

*Being back in control of my life and learning to accept
my new body is empowering. I am no longer afraid of my MS.
Yoga opened up my world and gave me purpose.*

MARY, YOGA MOVES STUDENT

Guiding Principles

Yoga Moves Philosophy

There is no single formula for practicing adaptive yoga. Healing is not necessarily curing a condition, physical ailment, or disease. Rather, it is a way to nourish the soul, while maintaining and improving your quality of life. *Adaptive Yoga Moves Any Body* is designed to cultivate your own healing power with a sense of playfulness and empowerment; uniting your mind, body, and spirit for an integrated practice. A renewed zest for living in the present moment with a sense of purpose and joy is within you.

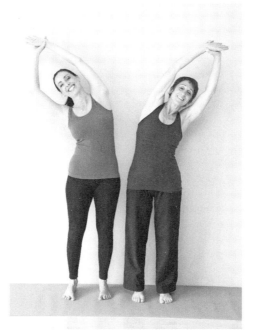

Be Playful

Leela is a Sanskrit word that translates into 'play', and that is exactly what adaptive yoga entails. Yoga is a way to feel alive and thrive in your body. It is much more than the physical postures. Yoga is about being creative, playful and spontaneous, on and off the mat, without expectations. It provides a release, and is known to improve immunity, stress, mood, pain, longevity, and relationships. Have fun with your practice. Laughter and giggles are good for your health. Smiling relieves tension in the jaw,

Guiding Principles

which can lead to more relaxed shoulders, hips and legs. Begin each practice by lifting the corners of your mouth for the most important pose in this book—a smile.

Enjoy Empowerment

The more you connect your mind, body, and spirit, the more you discover your capabilities rather than your disabilities. By harnessing your inner power, you can manifest changes you never thought possible. Saying, "Yes, I can" gives you empowerment. Saying "I can't" is obstructive. Even stating, "I am trying" doesn't show enough resolve. With a little faith in yourself, you can have more control over your body. This is summed up in the words of Yoda, the diminutive yogi from Star Wars, "Do or do not. There is no try."

Invite Healing

Everyone heals differently. Individuals with physical challenges, MS, neuromuscular, and immune conditions can benefit from a variety of healing approaches. Although there is no absolute path, you can invite healing into each day by integrating lifestyle choices with a comprehensive approach. Once Yoga Moves principles are applied on your yoga mat, you will begin to practice and benefit from them off the mat as well.

GUIDELINES FOR A HEALING PRACTICE

Prioritize Safety

The guiding yogic principle of *ahimsa* means to do no harm to yourself or others. Treat yourself sweetly. Refrain from a particular posture if it does not look or feel safe given your body's unique design and capabilities.

Be Mindful

Mindfulness is a process of awakening by intentionally paying attention to the here and now, inside and outside of you, throughout your day. Being present is an innate skill you already possess. Also known as

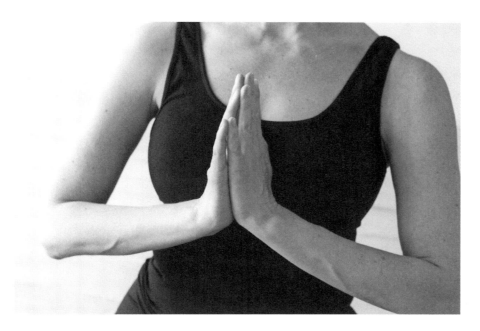

heartfulness, mindfulness includes the principles of non-judgment and acceptance. Accepting circumstances as they are is not the same as giving in to challenges. Apply mindfulness during your yoga practice by attuning to your breath, the sensations in your body, your thoughts, emotions, and reactions to them. Move with awareness, taking time to enter a pose. Allow the body to get to know itself through sensation. Be in the posture without rushing to get out of it. Feel the "echo" or impact as you exit a pose before transitioning to another.

Begin Your Practice With an Intention or Dedication

By setting a heartfelt intention or dedication at the beginning of your yoga session, you set a tone for healing and a purpose. This is called *Sankalpa* in Sanskrit. By dedicating your practice time to personal healing or to another person or concept in your thoughts, *Sankalpa* gives more meaning to life.

Seal Your Practice With Gratitude and Honor

At the conclusion of a practice, add meaning by acknowledging, honoring, and offering blessings to yourself, family members, friends, and your community. One of my favorite ways to end a practice is by

Guiding Principles

When yogic instruction rekindled a feeling of energetic sensation within my mind-body relationship, it felt like settling into a warm bath—the relief, the feeling of nourishment, the calm and quieting reference. I grew in dimension as my entire *body began whispering to me once again, albeit in a more eloquent voice.*

MATTHEW SANFORD,
*WAKING: A MEMOIR OF TRAUMA
AND TRANSCENDENCE*

saying the mantra, *"Lokah Samastah Sukhino Bhavantu,"* which translates to, "May all beings be happy and free." Another way you can complete your practice is by saying *"Namaste,"* which is a Sanskrit expression of gratitude, and acknowledges the light within all of us.

Respect and Honor Your Body

Help defray any anger or resentment you might feel that your body has betrayed you, by referring to your body parts as "co-workers". The intricate parts are working together, doing the best they can. Being in a body is a miracle, and each day it performs miracles that keep you alive. One of my favorite quotes by Jon Kabat-Zinn is, "as long as you are breathing, there is more right with you than wrong with you."

Balance Energy and Fatigue Through Breath

Yoga has a direct impact on *prana*, the Sanskrit word for life force or energy. Breathing exercises, physical poses and meditation have a high impact on your energy level, and are known to open the many energy channels throughout your body. Use your breath as an "edge detector" to learn your current capabilities. An erratic, uneven, or held breath is a sign that physical effort exceeded that edge. If your breath becomes irregular, a break is warranted. Taking a break means that you are paying attention to your body and allowing it to rebalance through a steady breath. The advanced yogi is not the one who can put their foot behind their head. It is the one who knows when to take a break.

Visualize Movement

If fatigue is high, or if a pose appears beyond your current capability, visualize yourself in the pose as if you were physically doing it. Scientific research shows that when this is done there is a physiological response, and the brain activates as if you were actually moving. Yoga Moves students report that they believe their toes are moving, no matter whether they can see it happening, or feel the sensation.

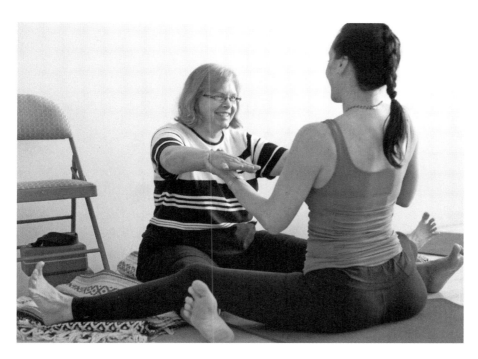

Know Sensation

Yoga helps you become aware of sensation. Individuals with MS and neuromuscular conditions often experience numbness, burning, tingling, or pain. Our instinct is to react to discomfort and pain by escaping or pushing the feelings away. This approach often leads to increased pain. Another coping strategy is to welcome any of these sensations, no matter how subtle. Even the absence of an expected sensation is a focal point for increased awareness.

All Gain with No Pain Yoga should not hurt, cause acute pain, or steal your breath. Yogis learn to distinguish sharp pain from mild temporary discomfort. If your discomfort or pain continues or increases, exit the pose gently and rest for a few breaths before continuing with a different action. Visualize your breath distributing nourishment to all parts and cells of your body to help diminish your focus on a specific area of pain.

Experience the Stretch Strike a balance between your excitement to increase flexibility and your caution due to fear of hurting an

Guiding Principles

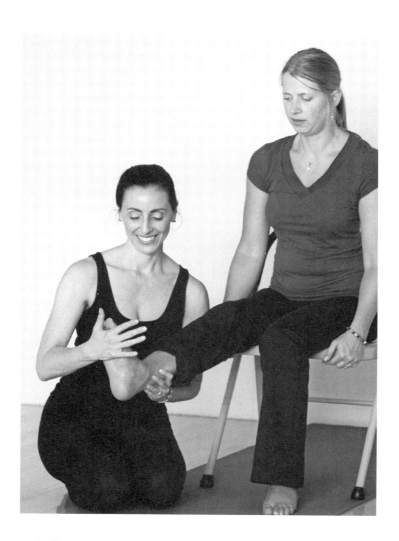

inflexible body. Yogis with hyper-mobility in the joints experience injury more frequently. Go slowly to explore your inner landscape and welcome your sensations. Many practitioners often do not feel the intensity of the stretch until a pose is held for several breaths. Begin by holding a stretch for 3 to 5 breaths and gradually increase the holding time to 10 to 15 breaths. If you notice you are holding your breath, you have stretched beyond your edge.

Spasms and Cramps Muscle spasms cause contractions and rigidity. While they are abrupt and uncomfortable, they provide sensations and important messages. Stretching to the point just before the spasm triggers is more effective than pushing too far toward another spasm. Spasms can teach you how far is too far, and where the stretch is just right. When a spasm does occur, ground the chaotic energy in the muscles by providing direction and a path for release. For instance, if you are in a chair, and your leg starts bouncing, press the thigh down with your hands to send the energy toward the earth. Or if you are lying down, you can extend your spastic leg and send the energy out through your heel. Alternatively, focus on your breath upon the onset of a spasm. Place a blanket under your hips, knees, ankles, or feet to prevent or lessen spasms if you notice they are triggered by touching the earth or mat. Additionally, sometimes placing a light weighted sand bag on the area quiets them.

Build Overall Strength Imagine a centerline running through your body from your crown to the bottom of your feet. When you pull your muscular energy inward toward this line, you are building strength from the periphery to the core. Visualize hugging your skin to the muscles, and your muscles to the bones. Pressing outward from your center also builds strength from the inside to outside.

Another way to build strength is with resistance. You can use the wall, the earth, a body part, or engage a yoga buddy to press against and provide leverage. For example, imagine pushing your feet down and away from you while seated or standing. Feel the sensation of tapping into your strength. Be cautious not to overdo because excessive effort can lead to rigidity. Likewise, too little effort, leads to instability. Core strength is specifically addressed in Yoga Moves Your Core (see page 88).

Sensory Awareness Draw your attention to physical sensations. You may alternate your focus on the sensations or areas of discomfort, with areas or sensations in the body that are pain free, to observe your thoughts, reactions and emotions. Then return to the breath as the anchor of awareness. Practice releasing any held pain or thought with each exhale.

Guiding Principles

*To let go means
to give up
coercing, resisting,
or struggling,
in exchange for
something more
powerful and
wholesome which
comes out of
allowing things
to be as they are
without getting
caught up in
your attraction
to or rejection
of them, in the
intrinsic stickiness
of wanting, of
liking and disliking.
It's akin to letting
your palm open to
unhand something
you have been
holding on to.*

JON KABAT-ZINN,
*WHEREVER YOU GO, THERE YOU
ARE: MINDFULNESS MEDITATION
IN EVERYDAY LIFE*

Refrain from a Results-Oriented Focus

Your yoga practice is not about success, failure, or perfection. Researchers may choose to focus on results. But you should concentrate on your present capabilities. Celebrate your efforts and successes of any measure or size.

Meditate Daily

One of the most powerful daily habits or rituals is meditation, which helps you gain, maintain, or reclaim a sense of wholeness. With meditation you can deepen and strengthen the relationship you have with yourself and others.

Many practitioners feel that they cannot meditate because their mind wanders, and they cannot sit still. The mind is acting as it should. The mind does wander, and being still is a challenge. Meditation is not easy, though the concepts are simple to understand.

There are many different ways to meditate. Experiment to determine which method works best for you. Most meditative techniques involve paying attention to your breath, either in the foreground or background of your thoughts. A simple meditation technique is to softly stare at a candle flame in a dimly lit room as you breathe consciously. By focusing intently on one simple thing, your thoughts can drift away as you become aware only of the candle flame.

You can use your breath to help you settle, while at the same time using simple words or a *mantra*. For example, practice "Letting Go." Breathe in as you say to yourself "let," and breathe out as you say to yourself "go," repeating these words with each breath for the duration of your meditation.

With formal mindfulness meditation, you use the breath to anchor your mind in the present moment. Learn to shape the quality of your life by noticing how you focus, sustain, and shift your attention with a beginner's mind. Consciously observe your thoughts, emotions, and reactions without trying to push them away or grasp onto them. It is common to be unaware of negative thought patterns that can diminish your quality of life. Allow the wave of emotions to come and go with this newfound awareness. Practicing loving kindness toward yourself and others helps to reverse or lessen these negative thoughts. Acknowledging and accepting them is required before they can be changed. As thoughts change, behavior changes, and the body adapts too. With compassion, open your heart to whatever there is to feel, from unpleasant to pleasant, from pain to joy, from fear to freedom, and from

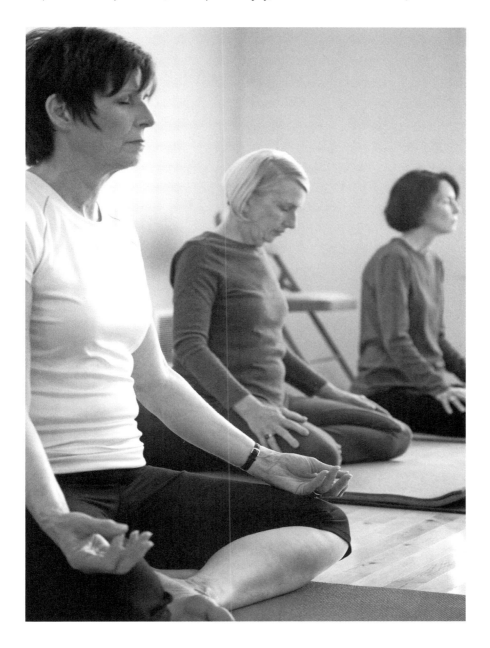

Guiding Principles

anger to love. Start your meditation practice with three minutes each day and gradually increase the time by a few minutes every week or month until you are able to sit for twenty or more minutes a day.

A body scan is often used to build the mind-body connection, and is a precursor or alternative to meditation. You can begin in a reclining or seated position, and sequentially direct your thoughts and breath to parts of your body, starting with your toes and directing your thoughts through your body to the top of your head. Notice your thoughts, emotions, and reactions. Over time, you may lead yourself through a personalized scan so that you can vary the time spent on parts of your body depending on your needs.

If you prefer a more active form of meditation, contemplative journaling can help you record your sensations. Write or type your thoughts, emotions, and reactions without lifting the pen from the paper, or your fingers from the keyboard. Afterwards, read what you have written, or not. If you choose to read, you may look for common patterns, themes, or words.

Serve Others

By the act of giving, you will receive tenfold the benefits of what you have given. *Karma Yoga* is about helping others and yourself by cultivating a sense of community, contribution, purpose, and gratitude. Examples of simple acts of kindness include smiling at a stranger, picking up litter on the street, buying or making a healthy smoothie for a friend, sending a thoughtful email to a lonely relative, or volunteering at a nearby senior center. Offer a *karmic* act of service to others at least once a day to stay in touch with humanity and heal yourself.

CHAPTER 4

*"I have found the breath to be one of the most fundamental
parts of yoga. The poses will not be as effective without the breath.
It is freeing in a spiritual way. MS may restrict your movements but not
the act of the breath. It can be learned and practiced at all times.
The breath is an excellent way to relieve stress."*

CARLA, YOGA MOVES STUDENT

Breath Practice

Pranayama

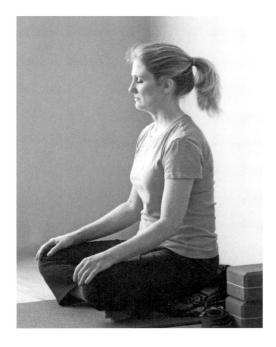

"Prana" means vital energy or breath of life. **"Yama"** means control of your breath experience. *Pranayama,* your breath practice, is essential to yoga. A breath synchronized with movement balances effort and ease. Holding your breath while concentrating can restrict benefits. Without attention to the breath, the poses are simply positions of the body and do not reflect the true potential of yoga to connect the mind, body, and spirit.

The qualities of the breath are experienced in terms of the rate, length, depth, sound, and sense of completion of the inhalations and exhalations. A natural, balanced breath is used during pose practice, and other breaths sampled here are used for different effects. The breath is both nourishing and cleansing. Each inhale brings fresh oxygen, and each exhale releases toxins from the body. A conscious, flowing breath contributes to a balanced nervous system and emotional state. It can either be deeply calming, or serve as a superpower energizer. In addition, when used in meditation, the breath is either in the foreground as a focal point or in the background as a centering force. Breathing is involuntary, but can be controlled. It is life sustaining.

Complete Yoga Breath

PRIMARY BENEFITS

- Yields a purifying effect
- Calms nervous system
- Prevents chest breathing and hyperventilating
- Provides focal point for concentration
- Lowers heart rate and blood pressure
- Massages and tones abdominal, pelvic floor, and spinal muscles
- Increases vital energy flow
- Can be practiced at any time and anywhere

PRECAUTIONS

- Nasal congestion

PROPS

- Yoga mat
- Chair
- Blanket
- Sandbag

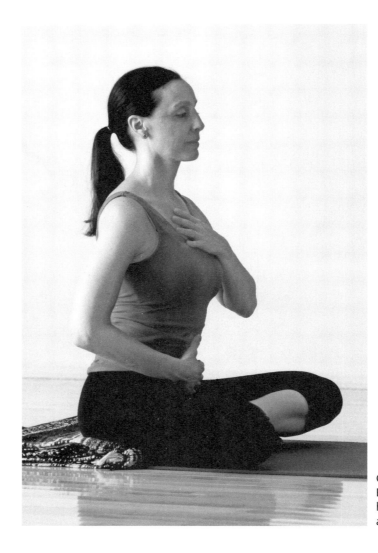

Complete Yoga Breath with hands on belly and heart

BREATHING INSTRUCTIONS

1. Begin in a comfortable seated position, either in Easy Pose or Mountain Pose in a Chair, OR on the earth in Bridge Prep Pose (see pages 175, 222, or 137, respectively, for instructions).You may rest both hands on your thighs, OR one hand on your belly and one hand on your heart. The lips gently touch OR have a little space between them. The jaw and the tongue are relaxed.

2. Observe your breath. Become attuned to the current quality of your breath without any judgment.

3. Concentrate on breathing from your belly.

4. Inhale through your nose and into the back of your throat. Observe your belly rising. Feel this expansion spread into your rib cage and up toward your collarbone as your chest lifts toward your chin. This is called diaphragmatic breathing.

5. Exhale through your nose, feeling the chest, front ribs, and belly recede like a wave. Moderate your inhales and exhales so they are equal in length.

6. Enjoy Complete Yoga Breaths, practicing 10 to 20 breath cycles.

7. Avoid gasping, pushing, or pulling the inhalations or exhalations.

8. Over time, gradually increase the repetitions and begin to lengthen the inhale and exhale breaths. You will learn to make your breath deeper, longer, stronger, and more productive.

ADAPTATIONS AND VARIATIONS

- When practicing on the earth, place a sandbag on your belly to help you feel the wave of the breath.

- Increase the length of an inhale to increase your energy and alertness.

- Increase the length of an exhale to reduce anxiety and tension, and improve restfulness.

I use yoga every night when I go to bed. My focus on breathing helps me fall asleep.

TERRI, YOGA MOVES STUDENT

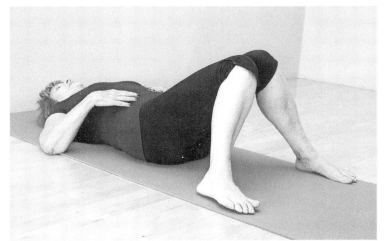

Constructive
Rest Pose

Complete Yoga Breath

Practicing 'Letting Go' has taught me to relax and free my mind and body.

- Gradually increase the duration of an inhalation and exhalation for up to 5 counts each. If you notice that either increasing the length of the inhalation or exhalation, or both, is increasing your level of anxiety, return to focusing on your natural breath without trying to extend it. Then slowly increase the counts of your respirations over time.

- Practice while standing in Mountain Pose.

- Practice in Constructive Rest Pose. Begin in Bridge Prep Pose. Widen your feet and let your knees fall toward the center, resting against each other. Place one hand on your belly and one hand on your heart.

- Practice "Letting Go." On an inhale say "let," and on an exhale say "go," and repeat for 3 to 5 breaths. You can also do this with a smile for an added calming effect!

Pursed Lip Breath

Kaki Pranayama

PRIMARY BENEFITS

■ Soothes nervous system and lengthens exhales

PRECAUTIONS

■ Nasal congestion

PROPS

■ Yoga Mat

■ Chair

■ Blanket

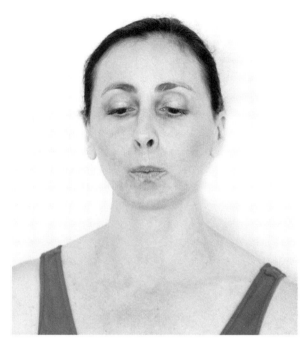

Pursed Lip Breath

BREATHING INSTRUCTIONS

1. Begin in a comfortable seated position such as Easy Pose or Mountain Pose in a Chair (see pages 175 or 222, respectively, for instructions).

2. Observe your normal breath and take 2 or 3 Complete Yoga Breaths.

3. Inhale deeply through your nose.

4. Purse your lips as if you were blowing out a candle, and exhale slowly for a count that is twice the length of your inhale.

5. Enjoy Pursed Lip Breath 3 to 5 times, inhaling through your nose and exhaling through pursed lips.

ADAPTATIONS AND VARIATIONS

• Practice standing OR on the earth.

Alternate Nostril Breath

Nadi Shodhana

PRIMARY BENEFITS

■ Calms and centers mind in present moment

■ Improves brain function

■ Balances nervous system

■ Produces optimal function to both right and left hemispheres of brain

■ Prepares mind for meditation

■ Improves relaxation and sleep

■ Regulates body temperature by balancing cooling and heating breaths

PRECAUTIONS

■ Nasal congestion

■ Anxiety or agitation with breath retention

PROPS

■ Yoga Mat

■ Chair

■ Blanket

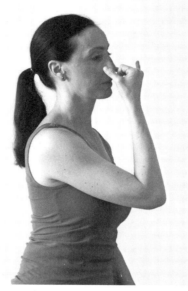

Alternate Nostril Breath with middle fingers in palm of hand

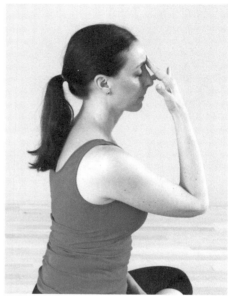

Alternate Nostril Breath with middle fingers at third eye

BREATHING INSTRUCTIONS

1. Begin in a comfortable seated position such as Easy Pose or Mountain Pose in a Chair (see pages 175 or 222, respectively, for instructions).

2. Keep a tissue handy for nostril cleansing before practice.

3. Take 2 to 3 Complete Yoga Breaths.

4. Fold your index and middle fingers of your right hand toward your palm, close the right nostril with your right thumb.

5. Inhale through your left nostril. Close your left nostril with your right ring finger, and simultaneously remove your right thumb from right nostril. Exhale through your right nostril.

6. Inhale through your right nostril. Then close your right nostril with your thumb, and simultaneously remove your ring finger from your left nostril. Exhale through your left nostril.

7. Inhale through your left nostril, then close it with your ring finger and release your thumb to exhale through your right nostril.

8. Repeat alternating sides. Notice on each side there is one exhale, then one inhale through that nostril, before alternating your breath on the other side.

9. Enjoy Alternate Nostril Breath for 3 to 10 breath cycles of complete inhalations and exhalations through alternate nostrils. Gradually work up to 3 to 5 minutes of daily practice.

ADAPTATIONS AND VARIATIONS

• Practice varying the length of your inhalations and exhalations. You can inhale for a count of 1 and exhale for a count of 2. Gradually increase the length at the same ratio, such as inhale for a count of 2 and exhale for a count of 4.

• Visualize alternating the breath through your nostrils without using your hands.

• Breath retention may be practiced by inhaling for a count of 1, retaining the breath for a count of 1, and exhaling for a count of 1. Use caution in proceeding with this practice if you are new to a breath retention practice; some people experience anxiety.

• Practice using the index fingers of each hand if you have limited finger mobility.

• Practice using the fingers on your left hand if you are left hand dominant.

• To help center yourself, place your index and middle fingers at your third eye instead of folding them in toward your palm.

I had vertigo and, for a medical test, I had to be off all my medications for 48 hours. My body was adversely reacting. My husband reminded me to use what I learned from my Yoga Moves class to help me. I made it though the is horrible time by meditating and doing Alternate Nostril Breathing... and lots of praying.

LYNN, YOGA MOVES STUDENT

⌇ *Cooling Breath*

Shitali

PRIMARY BENEFITS

■ Cools the body, and is highly recommended in hot weather or when body is hot

■ Reduces anger or agitation

PRECAUTIONS

■ Dizziness

■ Low blood pressure

■ Asthma or bronchitis

PROPS

■ Yoga Mat

■ Chair

■ Blanket

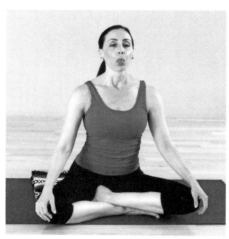

Cooling Breath inhale with curled tongue

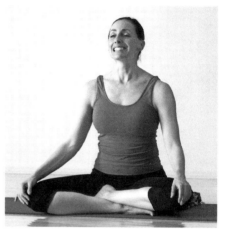

Cooling Breath option with upper and lower teeth closed and tongue tip on the roof of the mouth

BREATHING INSTRUCTIONS

1. Begin in a comfortable seated position such as Easy Pose or Mountain Pose in a Chair (see pages 175 or 222, respectively, for instructions).

2. Take 2 to 3 Complete Yoga Breaths.

3. Curl your tongue by bringing the sides of the tongue up toward the center.

4. Inhale through your curled tongue.

5. Relax your tongue, close your mouth and exhale through your nose. Repeat the cycle, breathing in through the mouth and rolled tongue, and out through the nose.

6. Enjoy Cooling Breath for 5 to 10 complete breath cycles.

ADAPTATIONS AND VARIATIONS

• The ability to curl your tongue is considered genetic. If you cannot curl your tongue in this manner, simply roll the tip of your tongue back to touch the roof of your mouth. Inhale through your teeth and exhale through your nose.

Lion's Breath

Simhasana

PRIMARY BENEFITS

■ Relieves facial and chest tension, sore throat, and bad breath

PRECAUTIONS

■ Practice in position that accommodates any knee condition, injury, or pain

PROPS

■ Yoga Mat

■ Chair

■ Blanket

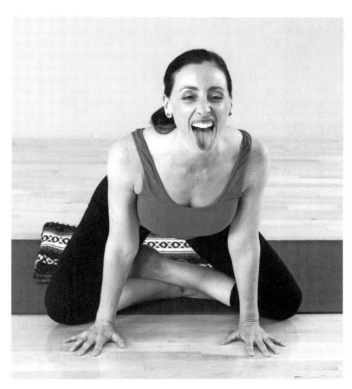

Lion's Breath leaning forward from Easy Pose

INSTRUCTIONS

1. Begin in a comfortable position such as seated in Easy Pose or Mountain Pose in a Chair, OR on hands and knees in Table Pose (see pages 175, 222, or 280, respectively, for instructions).

2. Take 2 or 3 Complete Yoga Breaths.

3. Inhale deeply through your nose.

4. Open your mouth wide, and stretch your tongue out as far as possible while making a "ha" sound, on a long exhale.

5. Enjoy Lion's Breath, roaring 3 to 5 times, inhaling through your nose and exhaling through a wide mouth, with tongue fully extended.

CHAPTER 5

"Yoga is so effective at strengthening, lengthening, and balancing the musculature and posture. But what yoga does for the mind and spirit is truly life shifting. When our body aligns in a balanced way, the energy flows through us with more ease, and the mind naturally aligns with its peaceful nature. Our spirit then seems to shine more palpably through our awareness and experience."

SARA DAVIDSON FLANDERS, YOGA THERAPIST

Alignment for Life

"Alignment for life" provides principles to help your body align optimally in yoga poses and throughout your day. Just sitting upright or standing mindfully are powerful yoga practices. As you become mindful of your alignment during yoga, you will also support your everyday movement patterns. Awaken your awareness of alignment while you brush your teeth, eat a meal, sit at your computer, in the car, on a train or plane, play a game or sport, watch a movie, and relax in bed.

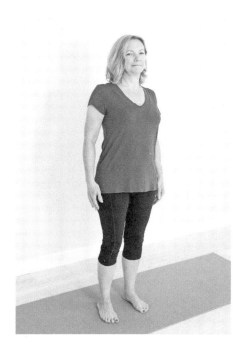

Properly aligned yoga poses help balance the musculoskeletal system. Attention to posture and the structural alignment of the body, together with conscious rhythmic breathing, can keep you safe and pain free.

You feel better, brighter, and lighter when you are aligned and energy flows freely through the body.

Alignment in an adult body is impacted by several factors, including genetic disposition, the way you move, and the environment. Since movement patterns are ingrained before you are necessarily conscious of them, considerable time is often required to modify habits.

When focusing on your body in relation to alignment, there is a tendency to be critical and expect perfection. Change in action is more important than form or appearance. Finding compassion, patience, and acceptance for the body's current physical state are essential.

Whenever you consider alignment to one part

Alignment for Life

Aligning the heart, mind, body and spirit does not alter the fact that you are facing challenges, but allows for a softening and possible dissolution of the tension and disappointment you may experience. Awareness and effort toward optimal physical alignment empowers you to access your optimal strength and spirit.

LYNN MEDOW, YOGA THERAPIST

of the body, it is helpful to look above and below the area of concern. Your body parts are intricately woven together. When one area in the body is adjusted and realigned, another area may be impacted. The more you practice yoga, the more you become aware of how movement and alignment impacts the whole body physically and energetically.

As you read and review the alignment principles and common tendencies, choose a focus. Perhaps, start from the bottom of your feet and work toward the top of your head. Or you may have one area of the body that is calling for attention. The general principles gradually absorb into the fabric of your tissues as muscles have memory. There is no need to force or push them into your body. To become conscious of a habit pattern is the first step toward change. Congratulate yourself for this realization.

You must consciously breathe for the duration of your practice, cycling rhythmically through each inhale and exhale, to help ease your progression through the poses. It is important to keep this rhythm and not hold your breath in concentration while entering a pose. Otherwise you will not receive the benefits of the pose and might even injure yourself.

This chapter explains alignment principles accompanied by common pitfalls. You are working toward the alignment described in the instructions, but don't worry if it is not accessible at first. Take small steps to assimilate the alignment concepts into your reality. For instance, if the instructions state to place the feet parallel in Mountain Pose, you may experience too much knee discomfort if you place your feet perfectly parallel, especially if the legs and feet are often externally rotated. A more feasible approach may be to start with a lesser degree of turnout, and then to make small movements toward parallel feet over several weeks or months.

Alignment is important from the crown of your head to the bottom of your feet and vice versa. Assimilating alignment principles into poses and daily movement patterns is a lifelong practice.

Foot and Ankle Alignment

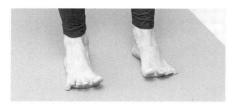

Feet aligned, toes lifted and spread

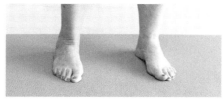

Feet parallel in "11"

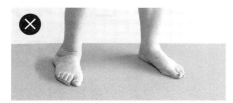

Weight on inside of foot, causing
ankle and knee misalignment

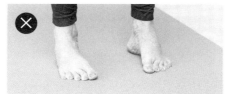

Weight on outside of feet, toes
crunched, ankles sickled

ALIGNMENT INSTRUCTIONS

1. Place your feet to form the number "11," or as close to parallel as you can comfortably manage. Turn the muscles and bones of your legs in the same direction as your feet.

2. Lift, lengthen, and spread your toes. Notice your arches also lift with this action. Keeping the tone in the arches, extend and lower your toes.

3. Press down evenly through the soles of your feet, with special attention to the center of the heels and the balls of your feet just below the big and little toes. These three pressure points form a tripod in each foot.

MISALIGNMENT CONCERNS

- Standing or walking with the feet in external rotation (turned outward). This can cause back and hip pain.

- Unevenly distributing weight in the foot, either with too much weight on the heel OR balls. This can cause weakness, alignment, and balance concerns in the feet, ankles, knees, and all the way up to the top of your head.

- Crunching or gripping the earth with your toes. This can make grounding difficult.

Knee Alignment

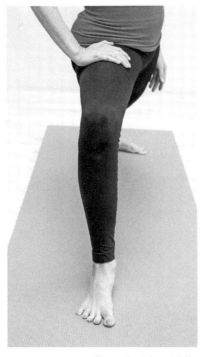

Knee aligned with middle toes, frontal view

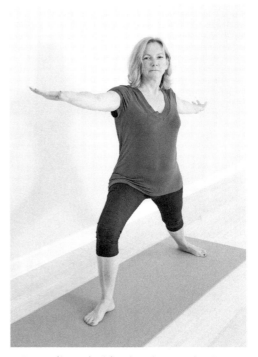

Knee aligned, side view in Warrior 2 Pose

ALIGNMENT INSTRUCTIONS

1. Maintain a slight bend in or soften your knee(s) when one or both legs are straight.

2. Align your knees with the middle toes so that your knees do not lean inward or outward.

3. In standing poses such as Warrior, stack your bent knees over your ankles and heels in standing poses. There are a few poses that are exceptions to this such as Crescent Kneeling Lunge, and Yoga Squat where it is safe to allow the knee to extend beyond the ankle because there is minimal weight bearing pressure on the bent knee. Be certain your knee aligns over your middle toes in these poses.

4. In seated poses such as #4, Firelog, or Butterfly, pull your knee to your chest and then rotate it outward to protect your knee.

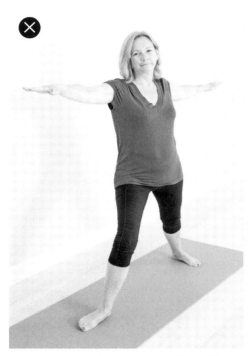

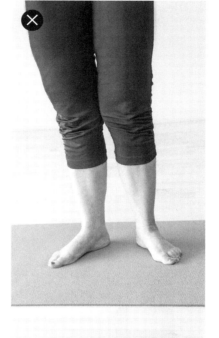

Knee caving in toward midline of body   Locked knees, feet turned outward

MISALIGNMENT CONCERNS

- Caving knees in or out from the center. This can cause pain and repetitive motion injury.

- Locking knee joints. This causes misalignment, inhibits balanced muscular action, and places unnecessary wear and tear on the joints.

- Moving knees past the toes in a bent leg pose. This puts too much weight on the joints, and can lead to increased risk of injury in poses such as Warrior Pose and Goddess Pose.

Leg and Hip Alignment Standing

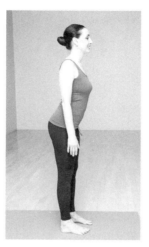 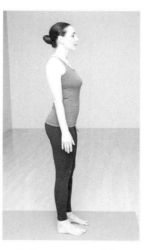 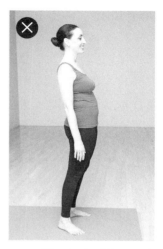

Thighs and hips moved back | Tailbone moved down and belly toned | Hips tucked forward, buttocks flattened and feet turned out

ALIGNMENT INSTRUCTIONS

1. Move your thighs and hips backward, and maintain unlocked knees. This action untucks your hips and pelvis.

2. Lengthen your tailbone toward your heels and pull your belly in and up. Tone the belly, buttocks, and pelvic floor muscles without gripping or squeezing.

3. At the same time, keep your ribcage level, rather than lifting the front ribs more than the back.

4. See Mountain Pose for additional instructions (page 220).

MISALIGNMENT CONCERNS – STANDING

• Thrusting hips forward, or tucking them under, often coupled with externally rotated feet. This can lead to slouching, imbalance, and back and hip pain, when the upper leg bones are not in the center of the hip socket.

• Unevenly distributing the weight on one leg. This forces the hip to the side and results in postural imbalance.

• Excessively squeezing the buttocks and pelvic floor. Constant muscle contraction can lead to weakness and tightness.

Leg and Hip Alignment Seated

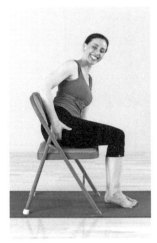

Moving flesh away from sitting bones

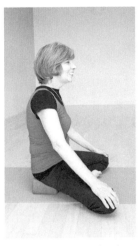

Neutral spine, seated on a block

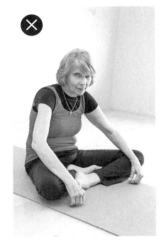

Back rounded back, "shlumpasana"

ALIGNMENT INSTRUCTIONS

1. Place a blanket or block under your hips if, when seated on the earth, your knees are raised higher than your hips. This will establish a neutral back curve. See Mountain Pose in a Chair for additional instructions (page 222).

2. Untuck your pelvis and hips, using your hands. Lean into your left hip, place your left hand on your inner right thigh and your right hand on your outer right hip. With the left hand turn the inner thigh muscles down and with the right hand move the flesh outward and back. Repeat on your left side.

3. Lengthen your tailbone down toward the earth and distribute the weight on your sitting bones.

4. Lift your ribcage and torso evenly toward your crown.

MISALIGNMENT CONCERNS – SEATED

- Rounding the lower back. This happens both if the knees are higher than the hips, and when slouching in "shlumpasana" posture. This leads to muscular imbalance between the front and back of the body.

- Excessively squeezing the pelvic floor. Constant contraction can lead to weakness and tightness.

🌀 *Spinal Alignment*

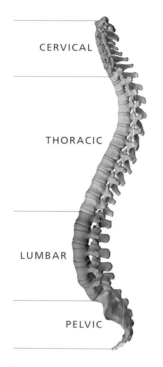

CERVICAL

THORACIC

LUMBAR

PELVIC

Spinal curves of vertebrae

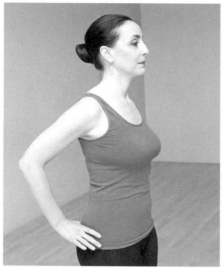

Ribs and belly pulled back and in

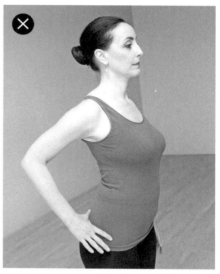

Ribs thrusted forward

ALIGNMENT INSTRUCTIONS

1. Focus on making space in the spine, from your tailbone to the top of your head.

2. Press down through your feet for stability and the energy will rebound to help lift your spine long and tall. This is known as the "root-to-rise" concept.

3. Pull your belly gently in and up toward your spine.

4. Lengthen the sides of the body by lifting up and out of the waist and breathing into the sides of your lungs. This creates space from the top of your hips to the middle of your armpits.

5. Lengthen the back of the body as much as the front.

6. Lift up through your crown and take several smooth Complete Yoga Breaths.

MISALIGNMENT CONCERNS

- Curving too much or too little at any of the spinal curves. The spine has four natural curves to absorb shock, and excess or minimal curvature disturbs optimal alignment.

- Collapsing torso inward, thrusting ribs forward, or scoliosis. These are examples of abnormal curves of the spine.

Shoulder Alignment

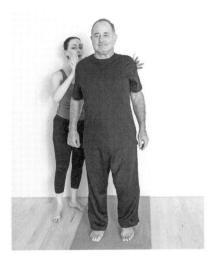

Drawing shoulder blades together onto the back

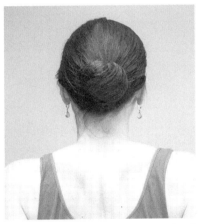

Shoulder blades on the back

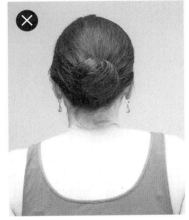

Pinched neck, rounded shoulders

ALIGNMENT INSTRUCTIONS

1. Shrug your shoulders up to your ears. Then drop them, letting them fall on their own. This calls awareness to the tension you may be holding in your shoulders

2. Lift your heart center, or sternum. Draw the shoulder blades together down the back, while keeping the chest and heart lifted. Refrain from squeezing the blades with too much intensity.

3. Broaden across the front of your body. The heart center, in yoga posture instructions, refers to the center of the chest, or the sternum, rather than the anatomical organ. Breathe into the heart center and across the collarbone.

Shoulder Alignment

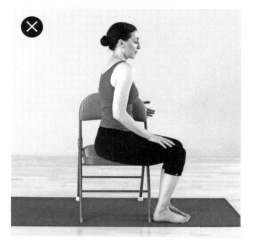

Seated with shoulders rounded and forward

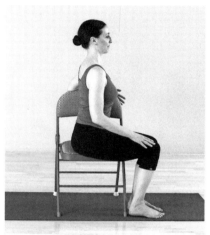

Seated with shoulders back

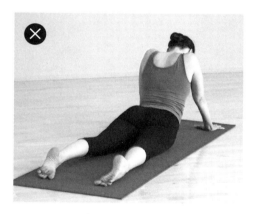

Hunched shoulders, head forward

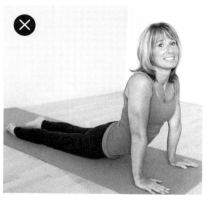

Locked elbows, shoulders forward

MISALIGNMENT CONCERNS

- Tightening shoulders. This can lead to tension in the facial, neck, and shoulder muscles.

- Slumping and rounding the shoulders. This can cause long term misalignment problems and occurs when the shoulders roll forward, collapsing the chest. I call this "shlumpasana." The rounded curve in the upper back can develop from natural aging, fatigue, depression, carrying heavy bags, and activities such as sitting in front of a computer screen or sinking into a comfy unsupportive sofa.

Head and Neck Alignment

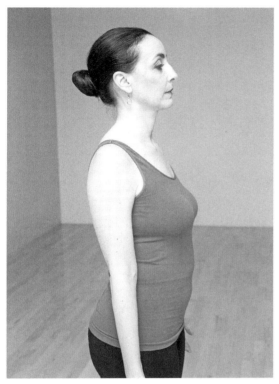

Neutral neck curve

The splendor and subtlety of living is most apparent in the conscious presence of the silence. Now, after thirteen years of yoga practice, not only do I feel an upward energetic release in hands-in-prayer, I also feel a downward energetic connection to the earth. Is this the same as being able to perform a complex, pretzel-shaped physical pose? Obviously not. Progress is what you make of it.

MATTHEW SANFORD,
*WAKING: A MEMOIR OF TRAUMA
AND TRANSCENDENCE*

ALIGNMENT INSTRUCTIONS

1. Balance your head over your tailbone.

2. Move your chin and soft palate back in space if your head is forward of your spine.

3. Lengthen your neck to make space between the vertebrae by rising up long through your crown (top of your head). The back of the neck should have a slight inward curve.

4. Refine how you hold your head with small adjustments. Move the top of your ears back, and tip your chin slightly down. The muscles on the sides of your neck should be soft and not overly worked.

5. Keep your gaze forward and level with the horizon. Where you focus your eyes impacts head and neck alignment and balance.

6. Relax the facial muscles and the tongue with space between your upper and lower jaw. Smiling helps.

Head and Neck Alignment

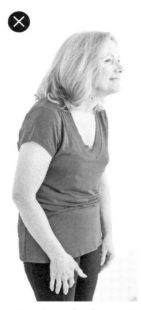 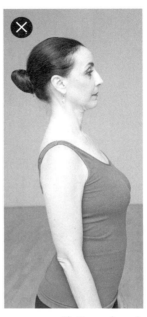 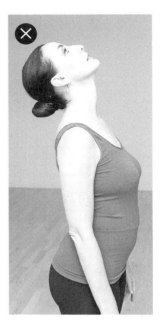

Head too far forward, rounded shoulders, and lifted chin

Flattened neck

Kinked neck

MISALIGNMENT CONCERNS

- Leading with the head, rather than the heart, as you move in space. This leads to rounded shoulders.

- Compressing or flattening the neck. This causes pain and can weaken the cervical spine.

- Curving the neck too far forward or backward. This strains the neck and leads to shoulder misalignment.

- Tensing the sides of the neck. This causes muscular imbalance.

- Jutting the chin forward and up, or tucking it in and down. This is often done in attempt to assume "good" posture, but it causes misalignment and discomfort.

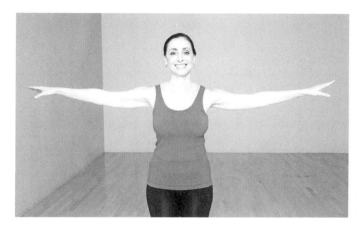 *Arms, Hands, and Wrist Alignment*

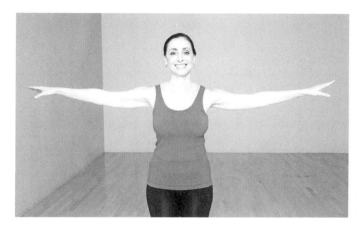

Energy extended through fingertips with arms in "T"

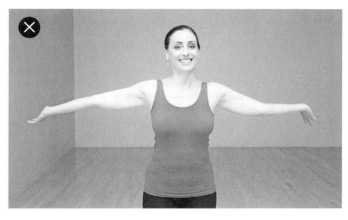

Right elbow locked, left wrist overly relaxed with arms in "T"

ALIGNMENT INSTRUCTIONS

1. Focus on a straight and energized arm.

2. In both weight bearing and non-weight bearing positions, maintain a slight bend in your elbows and draw your shoulder blades together down your back.

3. For weight bearing hand positions, press down firmly through the fingers and palms. Give special attention to the pads of your index fingers and thumbs as well as the roots of these digits, where they meet the palms. Spread the fingers and root their tips into the mat. Create balanced action across the hands and fingers.

4. For non-weight bearing positions, extend your arms outward from the heart through soft elbows, straight wrists, and fingers.

Arms, Hands, and Wrist Alignment

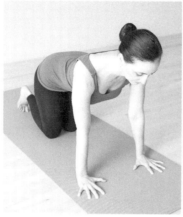 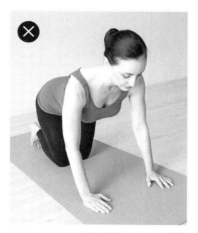

Fingers spread, tips pressing into mat, weight distributed across palms and fingers in Table Pose

Weight on outside of hands

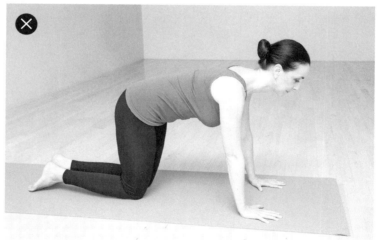

Locked elbows in Table Pose

MISALIGNMENT CONCERNS

- Locking the elbow joint. This makes the joint more vulnerable to injury.
- Placing weight on the outside of the hand or into the wrist, when in weight bearing poses. This action increases joint pain.
- Clenching or spreading fingers too far apart. This can cause over-exertion and tension.

🌀 Forward Bend Alignment

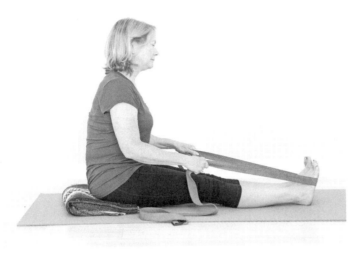

Forward Fold Pose at 90 degree angle, sufficient to feel the stretch

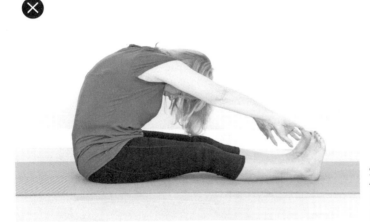

Struggling to reach toes in Forward Fold Pose

ALIGNMENT INSTRUCTIONS

Forward bends lengthen the back of the body and calm the nervous system. They are found in Forward Fold Pose, Pyramid Pose, Sage Pose and Stick Pose, among others.

1. Lengthen the spine and front of the torso while drawing the shoulder blades together down the back.

2. Hinge at the hips rather than at the waist, and move your spine toward your thighs.

Forward Bend Alignment

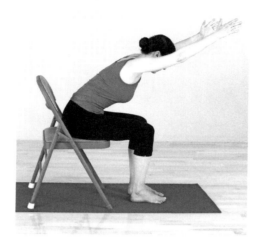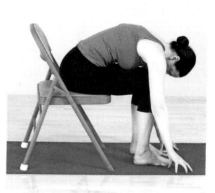

Forward Fold Pose in a Chair with shoulders on the back

Forward Fold Pose in a Chair with lengthened spine and shoulders rounded

3. Keep your hands near your hips, thighs, or shins, rather than struggle to reach your feet. Refrain from the urge to touch your toes. Finding length in the torso and back of the legs takes priority.

4. When fully in the pose, the shoulders may round as long as the lower back is straight and long, and is not rounded.

5. When in standing forward bends, you may soften your knees or bend them to touch your toes.

6. When in forward bends seated on the earth, elevate the hips to facilitate hinging at the hip joint and to lengthen the spine.

MISALIGNMENT CONCERNS

- Reaching too far to touch the toes. This can cause an overly rounded lower back and shoulders that can strain the back. Depending upon flexibility, the stretch can be felt with less of a bend.

- Bending at the waist rather than the hip joint. This causes rounding in the back.

- Locking the knees. This inhibits the upper and lower leg muscles from fully engaging.

☁ *Backbend Alignment*

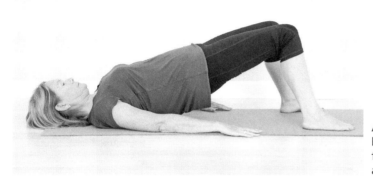

Aligned backbend, with feet parallel and long neck

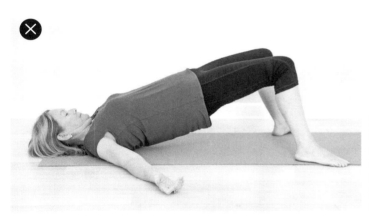

Misaligned backbend, externally rotated feet, tucked chin and compressed neck

> ❝
> *Through the regular practice of alignment in our body and mind we find our way to the Heart, the true source of health and peace.*
> ❞
>
> NATALIE PIET, YOGA THERAPIST AND AYURVEDIC PRACTITIONER

ALIGNMENT INSTRUCTIONS

Backbends are energizing and emphasize opening the heart and the front of the body. They are found in poses such as Bridge Pose, Camel Pose, Cobra Pose, Locust Pose, Sphinx Pose, and Thigh Stretch Pose.

1. Draw the shoulder blades together down the back.

2. Lengthen the tailbone, and tone the buttocks and the belly.

3. Engage muscular action in the legs and feet to keep grounded and prevent compression in the lower back.

4. Keep the front and the back of the neck long, and follow the curve in the spine created by the backbend.

Backbend Alignment

MISALIGNMENT CONCERNS

- Internally or externally rotating feet and clenching buttocks. This can lead to lower back and knee pain.

- Excessively curving the lower back and minimally curving in upper back. This can strain the back and create pain.

- Thrusting the hips or upper thigh bones forward in Camel Pose or upward in Bridge Pose. This can put unnecessary pressure on the lower back.

- Pushing the neck too far forward or backward, or flat. This takes the neck out of natural alignment with the spine.

- Pulling down the collarbone and ribcage toward the hips. This shortens the sides of body, decreases shoulder range of motion, and can cause tension in the neck and lower back.

- Rounding the shoulders, rather than drawing the shoulder blades down the back.

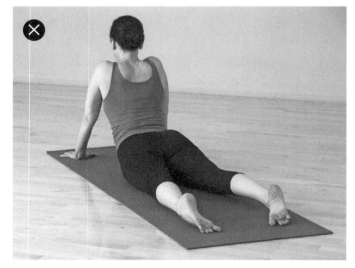

Hunched shoulders and crunched neck

⌇ *Side Bend Alignment*

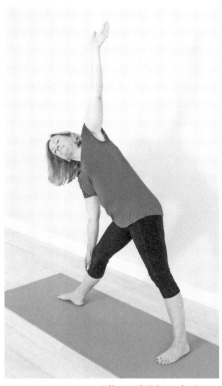

Aligned Triangle Pose

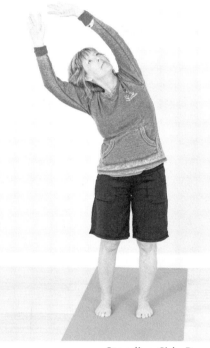

Standing Side Bend

ALIGNMENT INSTRUCTIONS

Side bends create an intentional curve in the spine toward one side at a time. They lengthen the muscles between the ribs and stretch the sides of the body. Triangle Pose and Extended Side Angle Pose are examples of side bends.

1. Pull your belly in and up to engage your core muscles.

2. Side bend to the right, and feel the stretch on the left side of the body. Repeat on the opposite side.

3. Bend in one plane with both sides of the body remaining long. Imagine you are practicing between two pieces of glass.

4. When side bending to the right, the left arm should lengthen over the ear, either skyward such as in Triangle Pose, or toward your crown in Extended Side Angle Pose.

5. Gaze up toward your arm, OR at eye level, OR down to the earth, depending upon your comfort.

Side Bend Alignment

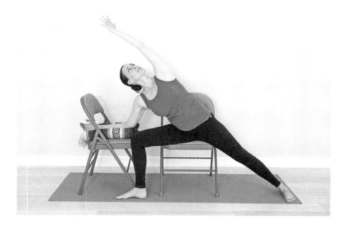

Extended Side Angle Pose with arm over ear

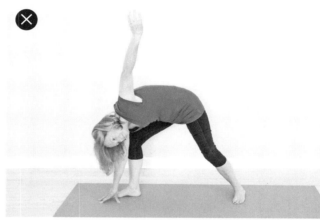

Arms Internally rotated, and torso stretched too far forward and down in Triangle Pose

MISALIGNMENT CONCERNS

- Bending forward while attempting a side bend.
- Leaning to the side without bending and engaging the core. This is not a true bend.
- Reaching too far down and forward. The benefits of a side bend are often lost to this misalignment.

〰 *Spinal Twist Alignment*

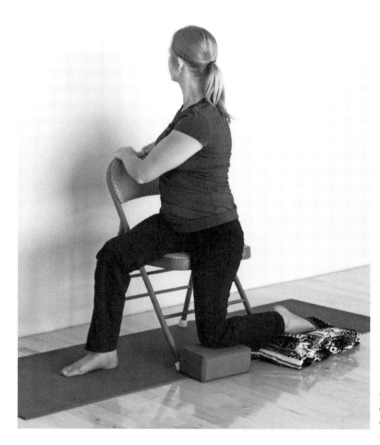

Spinal Twist
with pelvis
facing forward

ALIGNMENT INSTRUCTIONS

Twists increase and maintain flexibility in the spine, stimulate internal organs, and boost energy level in poses such as Reverse Triangle Pose, Sage Twist Pose, and Half Lord of the Fishes.

1. Create length from the base of the spine to the top of the head.

2. Rotate your spine to the right from your navel upwards. Turn your head last, to keep your head in line with your spine. Avoid over-twisting your neck.

3. Broaden across the heart and collarbone to open the shoulders.

4. Use your arms, hands, or fingers on a chair, the earth or your thigh for leverage.

Spinal Twist Alignment

5. In a seated twist on the earth, place a blanket under your hips to obtain a neutral lower back curve and prevent rounding.

6. In a standing pose, maintain a steady foundation with weight evenly distributed in the feet.

MISALIGNMENT CONCERNS

- Forcing the twist past your natural capacity. This can cause pain in the back or neck.

- Twisting the head and neck before twisting the lower spine. This can lead to straining the neck.

"The first thing I feel like doing in the morning is stretching my whole body by putting my arms above my head and taking deep breaths. Nothing feels better than that."

LORI, YOGA MOVES STUDENT

Warm Up, Tune Up, and Loosen Up

Don't let the phrase "warm up" scare you! Sweating is optional, but heating up to the point of exhaustion isn't the goal. Gain an awareness of your body, be amazed at what you can do, find space within, and be joyous in your movement. These are beginning exercises to help you feel safe, supple, strong and free.

"Warm Up, Tune Up, and Loosen Up" gives you instruments for your personal Yoga Moves toolbox. You may use these moves as stand-alone exercises, as precursors to your yoga practice, or in combination with a sequence of yoga poses. From head to toe, your entire body is covered in this section. Choose a daily selection of warm-ups that suit your needs and make you feel as though you

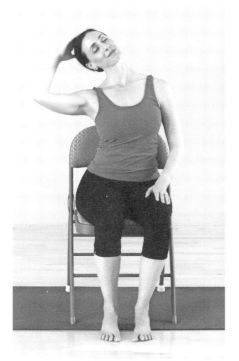

have bathed your whole body in movement.

These are introductory movements. Instructions for each start with a foundational pose found in the Yoga Moves "Adaptive Poses" chapter. Frequently, the beginning pose is some form of Mountain Pose. Instructions for asymetrical warm-ups are given to practice on the right side first. For balanced practice, repeat the instructions on the left side of your body. You will reap greater benefit from these warm-ups if you incorporate the alignment instructions provided in the foundational poses mentioned.

With these exercises you will build energy, strength, flexibility, and coordination. Let's get moving with a sense of safety, spirit, and fun!

🌿 *Yoga Moves Your Neck*

PRIMARY BENEFITS

- Builds neck strength
- Relieves tension
- Improves flexibility

PRECAUTIONS

- Spine, neck, shoulder, or elbow condition, injury, and pain

PROPS

- Yoga mat
- Chair
- Yoga block

How you hold your head impacts your inner beauty and outer presence. Be aware of the connections within your body from top to bottom and bottom to top, and everything in between. A dose of tender loving care combined with a smile and a giggle go a long way to keep the tension away!

The variations below may be practiced individually or in a sequence of your choice. Variations 1 through 3 are perfect antidotes to time spent in front of a computer.

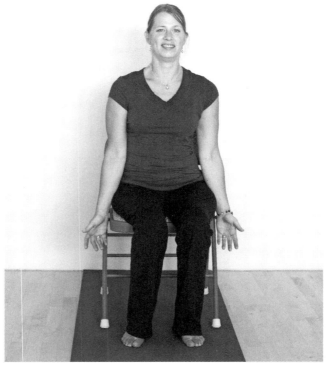

Mountain Pose in a Chair with arms at side and palms open

INSTRUCTIONS

Begin in Mountain Pose in a Chair (see page 222 for instructions) for Variations 1 through 3 and return to Mountain Pose between each neck release variation. Variation 4 is practiced on the earth. In order to benefit from these warm-up variations, begin in proper alignment. Awaken your spine and sit straight and tall.

VARIATION 1: SCALENE STRETCH

1. Begin in active Mountain Pose in a Chair with your spine straight and tall.

2. Place your right hand on top of your head.

3. Guide your right ear toward your right shoulder with your hand while keeping your shoulders level. Be careful not to dip your right shoulder as you do this.

4. You may change the stretch by varying your gaze skyward, OR eye level, OR to the earth, and by modifying the angle of your neck.

5. Enjoy Variation 1: Scalene Stretch on the right side for up to 3 breaths, and then lift your head back to center. To prevent over-stretching your neck, do not stay in the stretch longer than 3 breaths, and keep your heart center lifted.

6. Repeat the instructions above on the opposite side of your body.

7. Return to Mountain Pose in a Chair.

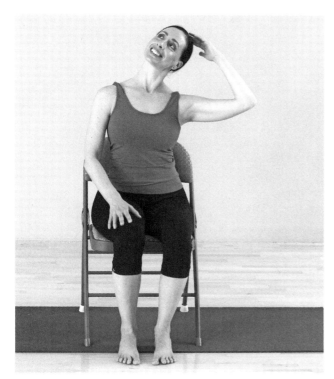

Variation 1:
Scalene Stretch
with gaze skyward

Yoga Moves Your Neck

VARIATION 2: CHIN TUCK

1. Begin in active Mountain Pose in a Chair with your spine straight and tall.

2. Exhale and lower your chin to your chest to lengthen the back of your neck.

3. Take one Complete Yoga Breath (page 28).

4. Inhale and lift your head to a neutral position with a forward gaze.

5. Enjoy Variation 2: Chin Tuck as you repeat 3 to 5 times.

6. Return to Mountain Pose in a Chair.

Note: Do not do this neck release variation if you have Lhermitte's sign.

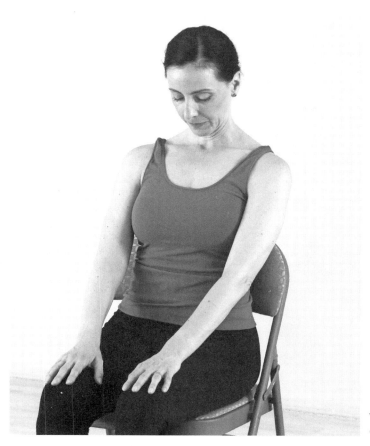

Variation 2:
Chin Tuck

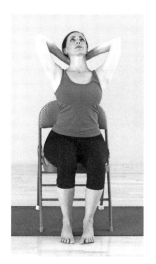
Variation 3:
Backbend

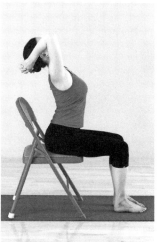
Variation 3: Backbend
in sideview

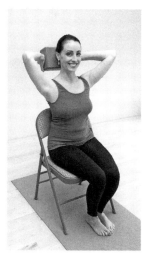
Variation 3:
Backbend with
block

VARIATION 3: BACKBEND

1. Begin in active Mountain Pose in a Chair with your spine straight and tall.

2. Interlace your fingers behind your head, cradling your lower skull at or below the occiput (the pointy part of your skull where a pony tail might be).

3. Support your head with your hands and draw your shoulder blades together down your back.

4. Lift your heart center skyward and tilt your head back slightly.

5. Apply gentle resistance as your head presses into your palms and your palms press into your head for a neck strengthener and lengthener.

6. Enjoy Variation 3: Backbend for 3 to 5 breaths.

7. Return to Mountain Pose in a Chair.

ADAPTATION TO VARIATION 3: BACKBEND

• Hold a block behind your head. Press your head into the block with your shoulder blades drawing together on your back.

Yoga Moves Your Neck

VARIATION 4: FISH POSE

1. Begin in Mountain Pose on the Earth, or Bridge Prep Pose (see pages 221 or 137, respectively, for instructions).

2. Place your arms into "robot" position with your elbows bent and your palms facing each other.

3. Press your elbows and the back of your skull into the mat as you arch your back off the mat.

4. Tilt your chin upward and lift your heart skyward, lengthening the front of your neck. Avoid rolling toward the top of your head.

5. Enjoy Variation 4: Fish Pose for 3 to 5 breaths.

6. Return to Mountain Pose on the Earth or Bridge Prep Pose.

 YOGA POSES TO MOVE YOUR NECK

See the "Index" to reference these sample poses to warm up, tune up, and loosen up your neck: Cobra; all Crescent poses; Locust; all Restorative poses; Table in Reverse. Be mindful of proper neck alignment in all twisting poses such as Half Lord of the Fishes, Sage Twist, and Thread the Needle.

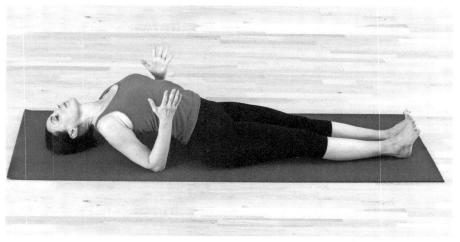

Variation 4: Fish Pose

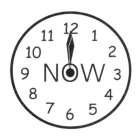 Yoga Moves Your Eyes

Eyes are said to be the window to the soul. Nurture your eyes and your soul with these Yoga Moves that you can enjoy throughout your day. The importance of exercising your eyes cannot be overlooked. (Pun intended!)

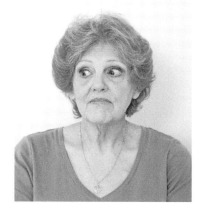

Eyes gazing at three o'clock

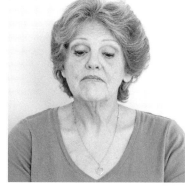

Eyes gazing at six o'clock

PRIMARY BENEFITS

■ Stretches eye muscles

■ Provides relief from gazing at electronic screen

■ Improves focus and concentration

PRECAUTIONS

■ Eye condition, injury, or pain

INSTRUCTIONS

1. Begin in Mountain Pose in a Chair (see page 222 for instructions) and imagine a large clock face in front of you.

2. Practice a Complete Yoga Breath (see page 28 for instructions) for 10 breaths with a soft gaze at the center of the clock.

3. Inhale and raise your eyes to gaze at twelve o'clock.

4. Exhale and return your gaze to the center of the clock.

5. Inhale and gaze at one o'clock.

6. Exhale and gaze back to the center of the clock.

7. Repeat this exercise and gaze at each consecutive hour in a clockwise movement. Match your breath with your gaze: inhale as you gaze at the hour on the clock; exhale and return your gaze to the center of the clock.

8. Repeat the exercise above in the opposite, or counterclockwise direction, matching your eye movements with your breath.

9. Soften your gaze and lower your eyelids half way to closing.

10. Enjoy this soft, unfocused gaze for 3 to 5 breaths to rest your eyes.

Yoga Moves Your Eyes

ADAPTATIONS TO YOGA MOVES YOUR EYES

- Move your gaze around the clock without moving your vision back to the center of the clock at each hour.

- Move your gaze to twelve o'clock. Take a Complete Yoga Breath. Move your gaze to six o'clock. Take a Complete Yoga Breath. Alternate moving your gaze up and down with your inhalations and exhalations, for three breath cycles. Then move your gaze to nine o'clock and take a Complete Yoga Breath. Move your gaze to three o'clock. Take a Complete Yoga Breath. Alternate moving your gaze side to side, inhaling and exhaling for three breath cycles.

- Throughout the day, frequently vary your vision field from objects close up, such as a computer screen, to objects in the middle distance approximately 20 to 50 feet away, and to objects in the far distance. For those who spend many hours in front of a screen, it is important to exercise your eyes in this way.

- When practicing yoga postures, notice how your gazing point affects your energy, balance, and tranquility. In particular, focusing on a small stationary object or point in front of you can aid in balancing positions.

🪷 *Yoga Moves Your Arms and Shoulders*

PRIMARY BENEFITS

▪ Relieves tension

▪ Improves range of motion in arms and shoulders

▪ Improves posture

PRECAUTIONS

▪ Shoulder, rotator cuff, or wrist condition, injury, or pain

PROPS

▪ Yoga mat

▪ Chair

▪ Yoga block

▪ Yoga strap

▪ Wall

No need to carry the weight of the world on your shoulders. Open your heart and tap into your strength.

Arm and shoulder openers benefit not only your shoulders, but also your head, neck, heart center, elbows, wrists, and hands. The variations below may be practiced individually or in a sequence of your choice. Although the variations are presented in a chair, they may be practiced standing or seated on the earth. You may wish to initially practice a few of the warm-ups facing a mirror to see that your shoulders are level.

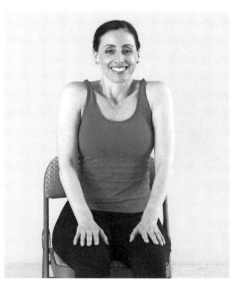

Variation 1:
Shoulder Circles

INSTRUCTIONS

Begin Variations 1 through 6 in active Mountain Pose in a Chair (see page 222 for instructions), and Variations 7 through 9 standing.

VARIATION 1: SHOULDER CIRCLES

1. Begin in active Mountain Pose in a Chair with your spine straight and tall.

2. Place your hands on your thighs.

3. Circle your shoulders up, back, down, and forward for 3 to 5 repetitions. These shoulder rolls are a nourishing self-massage.

4. Enjoy Variation 1: Shoulder Circles.

Yoga Moves Your Arms and Shoulders

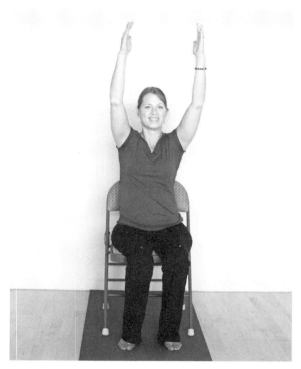

Variation 2:
Arm Lift

VARIATION 2: ARM LIFT

1. Begin in active Mountain Pose in a Chair with your spine straight and tall.

2. Turn your palms away from your body. Inhale, and slowly circle your arms skyward like they are moving through warm water or maple syrup.

3. Actively press your feet into the earth.

4. Lift your heart center skyward and draw your shoulder blades together down your back.

5. Keep your arms lifted for 3 to 5 breaths.

6. Turn your palms away from each other. Exhale, and slowly lower your arms down by your sides through the warm water or maple syrup.

7. Enjoy Variation 2: Arm Lift by following the instructions above for 3 to 5 repetitions, matching your movement to your breath. Lift arms as you inhale and lower arms as you exhale.

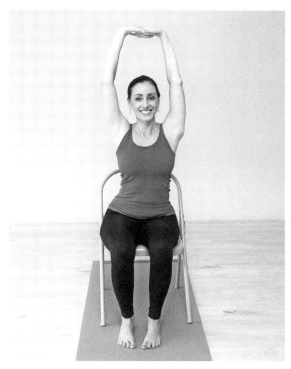

Variation 3:
Fingers Interlaced

VARIATION 3: FINGERS INTERLACED

1. Begin in active Mountain Pose in a Chair with your spine straight and tall.

2. Inhale and lift your arms straight in front of you at chest height.

3. Interlace your fingers and turn your palms away from you. Plug your arm bones into your shoulder sockets.

4. Raise your straight arms skyward while pressing your feet into the earth. Work toward aligning your elbows next to your ears.

5. Lift your heart center skyward and draw shoulder blades together down your back.

6. Enjoy Variation 3: Fingers Interlaced for 3 to 5 breaths.

Yoga Moves Your Arms and Shoulders

VARIATION 4: PALMS TO BLOCK

1. Begin in active Mountain Pose in a Chair with spine straight and tall.

2. Place a block between your hands. Press your palms into the sides of the block.

3. Inhale and lift your arms straight in front of you at chest height.

4. Exhale and press your palms into the block. Draw your arm bones into your shoulder sockets.

5. Inhale and lift the block skyward with straight arms.

6. Draw your shoulder blades together onto your back.

7. Exhale and lower the block to chest height while maintaining straight arms.

8. Enjoy Variation 4: Palms to Block for 3 to 5 repetitions.

ADAPTATION TO VARIATION 4: PALMS TO BLOCK

• Practice Yoga Moves Your Core, Abdominal Core Builders, Variation 3: Arm Lift (see page 91 for instructions).

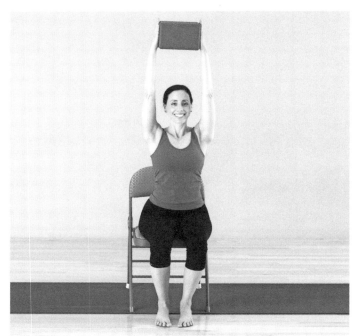

Variation 4:
Palms to Block
with straight
arms overhead

VARIATION 5: TO a "T"

1. Begin in Mountain Pose in a Chair with spine straight and tall.

2. Open your arms into a "T" with your palms facing skyward, OR to the earth.

3. Draw your shoulder blades together onto your back, broaden your collarbone, and soften the sides of your neck.

4. Reach out through your fingertips. This is a very subtle movement. Imagine a line of energy drawing out from your heart center into your fingertips. You will feel a sense of expansiveness.

5. Reverse the action and pull in on the same line of energy from your fingertips to your heart center.

6. Repeat this gentle energetic pulsation of drawing energy out to your fingertips and in toward your heart center.

7. Enjoy Variation 5: To a "T" for 3 to 5 breaths.

8. Release your arms to your sides.

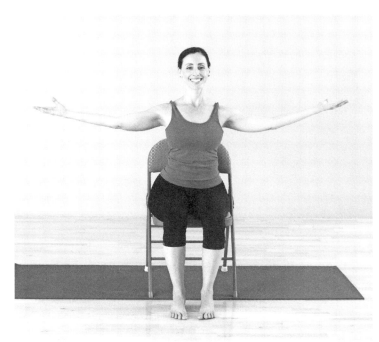

Variation 5:
To a "T"

Yoga Moves Your Arms and Shoulders

VARIATION 6: STRAP HAPPY

1. Begin in active Mountain Pose in a Chair with spine straight and tall.

2. Choose to use one of three strap options and follow the instructions:

   a. Make a loop with the strap that measures the width of your shoulders. Place the strap around your wrists. Lift your arms skyward in line with your ears, and with your palms facing toward each other. Press outward on the strap with your wrists or forearms. OR,

   b. Make a large loop with the strap that measures wider than your shoulders. Place the strap around your wrists. Forming a "V," lift your arms skyward in line with your ears. Press outward on the strap with your wrists or forearms. OR,

   c. Hold the strap firmly between your hands without clenching your fists. Position your hands wider than your shoulders to make a "V" with your arms. Lift your arms skyward in line with your ears. Pull your hands away from each other to make the strap tight.

3. With raised arms, draw your shoulder blades together down your back.

4. Feel the strength in your arms as you pull them away from each other.

5. Enjoy Variation 6: Strap Happy for 3 to 5 breaths and return your hands to your lap.

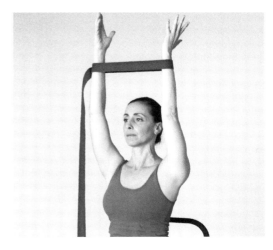

Variation 6: Strap Happy with strap around wrists, shoulder distance apart

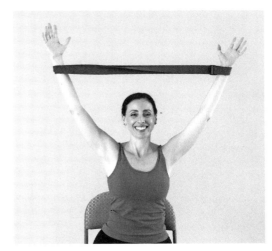

Variation 6: Strap Happy with strap around wrists, arms spread in "V"

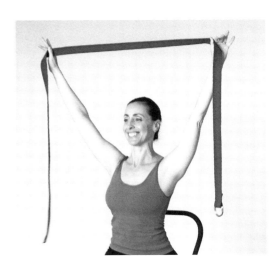

Variation 6: Strap Happy holding strap, and arms in "V"

Yoga Moves Your Arms and Shoulders

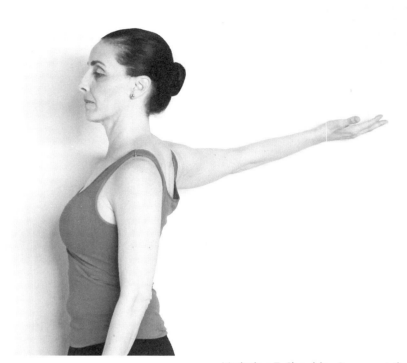

Variation 7: Shoulder Opener at the Wall, standing with palm skyward

VARIATION 7: SHOULDER OPENER AT THE WALL

1. Begin standing and face the wall.

2. Place your left hand on your hip. Raise your right arm to the side, placing your right hand on the wall slightly higher than shoulder height.

3. Plug your right arm bone into your shoulder socket. Draw both shoulder blades together down your back.

4. Lift both sides of your waist to lengthen your torso.

5. Turn your body away from the wall and toward your left, until you feel a stretch across your right shoulder. Take care to turn your neck last and keep it in line with your spine. If you feel any tingling or numbness, you may have turned too far. Release your arm and gently shake it.

6. Enjoy Variation 7: Shoulder Opener at the Wall for 3 to 5 breaths.

7. Repeat the instructions above using the opposite side of your body.

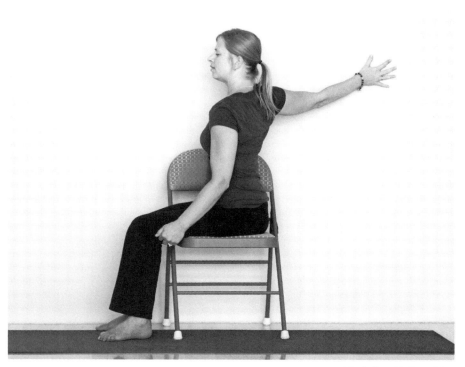

Variation 7: Shoulder
Opener at the Wall, seated

ADAPTATIONS TO VARIATION 7: SHOULDER OPENER AT THE WALL

- Practice seated sideways in a chair next to the wall, with your right side facing the wall.
- Use a "spider" hand with hand cupped and finger tips pressing into the wall.
- Practice with palm facing skyward and pinky finger pressing into wall.
- Angle your arm higher OR lower on the wall.
- Bend your elbow to feel a different stretch.

Yoga Moves Your Arms and Shoulders

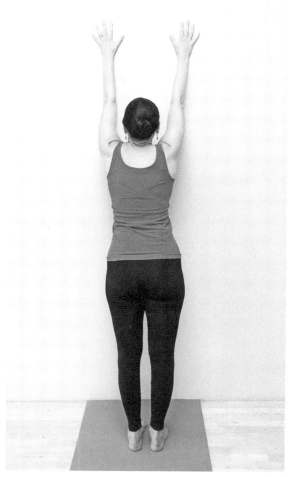

Variation 8:
Shower Pose
standing

VARIATION 8: SHOWER POSE

1. Begin in Mountain Pose facing the wall and positioned about a foot away from the wall (see page 220 for instructions).

2. Walk your hands up the wall until they are above your shoulders, or even above your head. Stop walking them up the wall when you begin to feel a stretch in your shoulders.

3. Press your hands into the wall and pull them energetically down toward the earth.

4. Draw your shoulder blades together onto your back.

5. Enjoy Variation 8: Shower Pose for 3 to 5 breaths.

ADAPTATIONS TO VARIATION 8: SHOWER POSE

- Place a chair next to you for support.
- Practice Shower Pose with a block between your thighs.
- Practice with heels lifted.
- Practice Cat and Cow Poses while standing in Shower Pose (see page 146 for instructions).
- Practice seated in a chair, facing the wall.
- Warm up your fingers at the same time with these "Finger Steps:"

  1. Walk one hand up the wall at a time, with each finger taking a step. Begin with your thumb and consecutively walk your index finger, middle finger, ring finger, and pinky finger higher on the wall, one "finger step" at a time.

  2. Once one hand has walked to the highest most comfortable position on the wall, repeat the exercise with your other hand.

  3. Walk each hand down the wall, reversing the order of fingers used as they step down.

The best and most beautiful things in the world cannot be seen or even touched – they must be felt with the heart.

HELEN KELLER

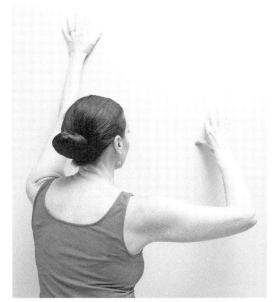

Variation 8: Shower Pose with Finger Steps on the wall

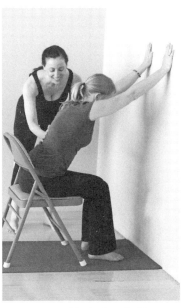

Variation 8: Shower Pose in a chair

Yoga Moves Your Arms and Shoulders

VARIATION 9: SCHLUMPASANA REMEDY

Too often we fall into a slouching posture both during our practice and throughout the day. The instructions below help to draw awareness to good shoulder and spinal alignment. You can practice this at any time as an alignment reminder, OR as a support when doing poses, OR when you go about your daily routine at home. You'll be surprised how good it feels!

1. Place a yoga strap at the base of your shoulder blades.
2. Bring the ends of the strap forward around your rib cage under your arms.
3. Toss the ends of the strap over each shoulder.
4. Cross the strap behind you to make an "X" on your back.
5. Grasp the ends of the strap near your hips.
6. Gently tug on the ends of the strap to tighten the harness and support your posture.
7. Enjoy Variation 9: Schlumpasana Remedy for 3 to 5 breaths, or as long as you want. You may also tie the strap around the front of your ribs to free your hands for other poses or activities.

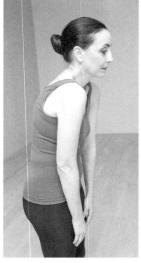
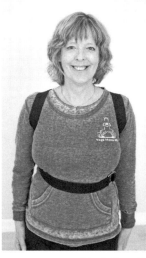
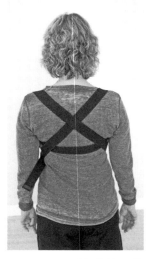

Variation 9:
Schlumpasana

Variation 9:
Schlumpasana Remedy
with strap, front view

Variation 9:
Schlumpasana Remedy
with strap, back view

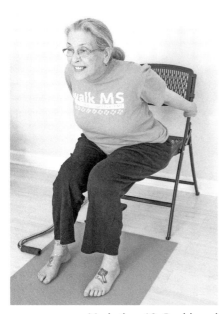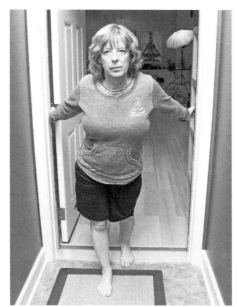

Variation 10: Backbend
Shoulder Opener in Chair

Variation 10: Backbend Shoulder
Opener in Doorway

VARIATION 10: BACKBEND SHOULDER OPENERS

- Begin seated, reach behind you and grasp the back of your chair. Lengthen the sides of your body and draw your shoulder blades together down your back. Lean forward, lift up through your heart center and enjoy this shoulder-opening backbend for 3 to 5 breaths. OR,

- Stand in a doorway and grasp the molding with your hands at about waist level. Lengthen the sides of your body and draw your shoulder blades together down your back. Take a step forward and lean away from the door jam until you feel a shoulder stretch. Enjoy for 3 to 5 breaths.

 ## YOGA POSES TO MOVE YOUR ARMS AND SHOULDERS

See the "Index" to reference these sample poses to warm up, tune up, and loosen up your arms and shoulders: Bridge; Camel; Child's; Cat and Cow; Downward Facing Dog; Cobra; Eagle; Headstand; Locust; Puppy; Sphinx; and Thread the Needle.

☙ *Yoga Moves Your Hands and Wrists*

PRIMARY BENEFITS

▨ Builds strength and flexibility in hands, wrists, and fingers

▨ Improves coordination

PRECAUTIONS

▨ Hands, wrist, finger injury, or pain

PROPS

▨ Chair

You hold the world in your hands: they can express; they can greet; they can massage; they can give and receive; they can be held. Hand and wrist releases are helpful to release the effects of repetitive tasks throughout the day. Try each variation here to see which helps you the most, OR alternate practicing different hand and wrist release variations.

INSTRUCTIONS

Begin Hand and Wrist Release Variations 1 to 6 in active Mountain Pose in a Chair (see page 222 for instructions), with your spine straight and tall. Begin Variation 7 in Forward Fold Pose in a Chair (see page185 for instructions).

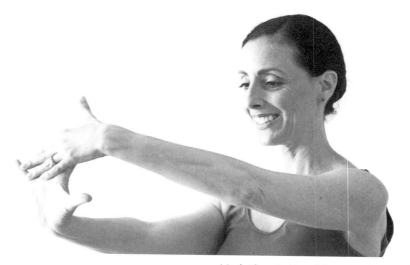

Variation 1: Hand Press Wrist Release

VARIATION 1: HAND PRESS WRIST RELEASE

1. Straighten your right arm in front of you at chest height, with your palm facing away from you, and spread your fingers and thumb wide.

2. Press the fingers of your left hand into your right fingers and palm. Feel the stretch across your right hand, wrist, and thumb.

3. Enjoy Variation 1: Hand Press Wrist Release for 3 to 5 breaths.

4. Repeat the instructions above using the opposite hands.

VARIATION 2: JULIE'S HAND AND WRIST RELEASE

1. Place your right hand in front of you at chest height, position the palm of your right hand facing left, and spread the fingers of your right hand.

2. Now, with the assistance of your left hand, slowly turn your right palm in toward your chest and beyond to face right.

3. Hold Variation 2: Julie's Hand and Wrist Release for 3 to 5 breaths.

4. Repeat the instructions above using the opposite hands.

Our warm-ups are very casual and a great way to shake off the cares and weights of the day.

DAVID, YOGA MOVES STUDENT

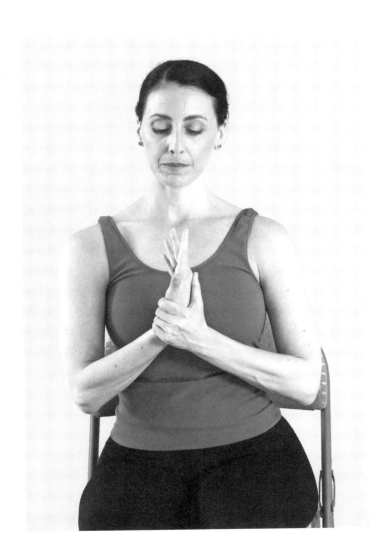

Variation 2:
Julie's Hand and
Wrist Release

Yoga Moves Your Hands and Wrists

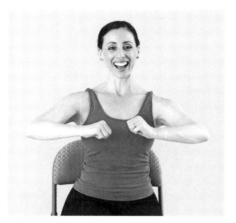
Variation 3: Wrist Circles 1

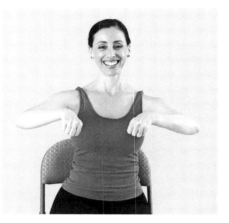
Variation 3: Wrist Circles 2

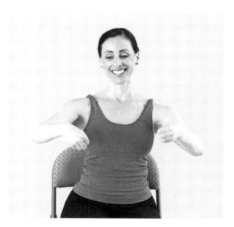
Variation 3: Wrist Circles 3

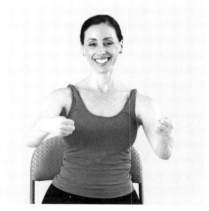
Variation 3: Wrist Circles 4

VARIATION 3: WRIST CIRCLES

1. Make a gentle yoga fist by placing your thumbs inside your palms and wrapping your fingers around the thumbs. Do not squeeze your thumbs.

2. Circle both of your wrists 3 to 5 times clockwise with your breath.

3. Circle both of your wrists 3 to 5 times counterclockwise with your breath.

4. Enjoy Variation 3: Wrist Circles, and feel the stretch across the top of your hands.

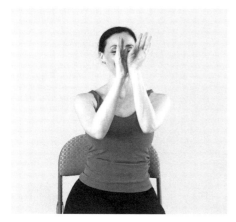

Variation 4: Candle Flame
Wrist Release 1

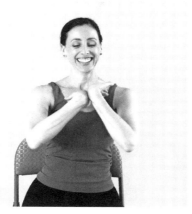

Variation 4: Candle Flame
Wrist Release 2

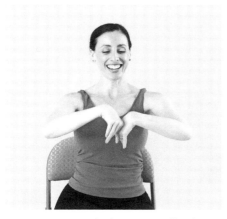

Variation 4: Candle Flame
Wrist Release 3

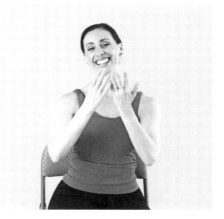

Variation 4: Candle Flame
Wrist Release 4

VARIATION 4: CANDLE FLAME WRIST RELEASE

1. Place your hands back to back.

2. Circle your hands around each other. The back of your hands or palms touch while fingers are free.

3. Have fun making different wave patterns with your hands for 3 to 5 breaths.

4. Repeat the instructions for Variation 4: Candle Flame Wrist Release above, circling your hands around each other in the opposite direction.

Yoga Moves Your Hands and Wrists

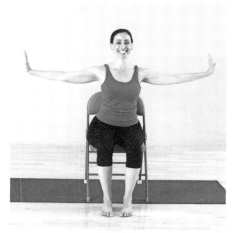 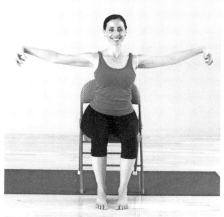

Variation 5: Wrist Flexion   Variation 5: "The Claw"

VARIATION 5: WRIST FLEXION

1. Lengthen your arms into a "T."

2. Flex your wrists and push your palms away from you, with your fingers skyward.

3. Draw your shoulder blades together on your back.

4. Next, curl your fingers under your wrists, while pressing your wrists away from you and keeping your fingers separated. This is known as "The Claw."

5. Repeat the flex and curl of Variation 5: Wrist Flexion 3 to 5 times with your breath.

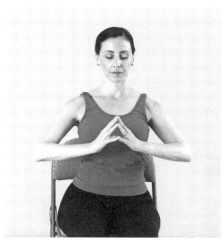

Variation 6: Spider Hand Push-Ups
with fingertips pressing
into each other

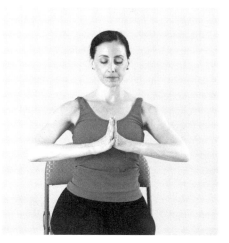

Variation 6: Spider Hand Push-Ups
with fingers pressing into each other

VARIATION 6: SPIDER HAND PUSH-UPS

1. Press your hands together in front of your heart center in a prayer position.

2. Draw your shoulder blades together down your back.

3. Pull your palms away from each other, but keep your fingertips touching.

4. Press the fingertips together of your right and left hands, applying equal pressure from your right and left sides.

5. Now allow the full length of the fingers on your right and left hands to touch together, keeping only your palms apart. Apply equal pressure along the length of your fingers.

6. Enjoy opening and closing hands in Variation 6: Spider Hand Push-Ups for 3 to 5 repetitions, following your breath.

Yoga Moves Your Hands and Wrists

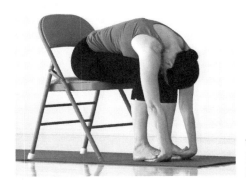

Variation 7: Hand-Under-Foot Release

VARIATION 7: HAND-UNDER-FOOT RELEASE
PADAHASTASANA

1. Begin in Forward Fold Pose in a Chair (see page 185 for instructions).

2. Slide your hands under your feet. Your palms are touching the soles of your feet and your toes are touching your wrist creases.

3. Gently press down with your feet onto your palms. The pressure against the hands should come primarily from the toes pressing into the wrist creases.

4. Enjoy Variation 7: Hand-Under-Foot Release for 3 to 5 breaths. You may also practice this wrist release in a standing forward fold position.

Note: Only do this wrist release if you can comfortably fold forward in a chair, OR from a standing posture.

 YOGA POSES TO MOVE YOUR HANDS AND WRISTS

See the "Index" to reference these sample poses to warm up, tune up, and loosen up your hands and wrists: Cobra; Downward Facing Dog; Handstand; Plank; Scale; and Table Pose variations. The spine is fundamental to all movement. Almost any yoga posture will strengthen your spine. It is important, however, to use your spine in a balanced manner, paying equal attention to moving it forward and backward, side to side, and twisting left and right.

Yoga Poses Move Your Spine

YOGA POSES TO MOVE YOUR SPINE

Warm-ups for your spine are found in many poses. See the "Index" to reference these sample poses to warm up, tune up, and loosen up your spine: Camel; Cat and Cow; Child's; Cobra; Downward Facing Dog; Forward Fold; Half Lord of the Fishes; Happy Baby; Inchworm; Locust; Mountain; all Restorative poses; Sage Twist; Spinal Balance; Spinal Twist; and Triangle. Also see Yoga Poses to Move Your Sides Variations.

> *Neurological deficit is a frontier of mind-body connection. Working with (my) students has taught me that the principles of yoga are nondiscriminating – they can travel through any body.*

MATTHEW SANFORD,
*WAKING: A MEMOIR OF TRAUMA
AND TRANSCENDENCE*

Yoga Moves Your Core

▧ Builds strong
central core

▧ Increases vitality and
inner strength

▧ Improves pelvic
floor function

▧ Relieves lower back
and pelvic pain

▧ Supports bowel,
bladder, and sexual
function

PRECAUTIONS

▧ Jaw, neck, spine, or
pelvic condition, injury,
or pain

PROPS

▧ Yoga mat

▧ Yoga block

▧ Chair

▧ Blanket

Many idioms such as "the fire in your belly" and having a "gut instinct" refer to the innate power in your abdomen. Stoke your inner fire for greater physical and emotional health. Tap into your inner strength and shine out from your center by combining the variations below.

This section focuses on two primary muscles groups for core building warm-ups: the abdominal and pelvic floor muscles. The abdominals work together with the back muscles to provide stability and balanced movement. The pelvic floor muscles at the root of your spine are indicative of your inner vitality, and they provide a protective hammock to support many essential organs.

Focusing on the abdomen and pelvic floor separately is often helpful to draw greater awareness to the individual muscle groups. First, practice the abdominal and pelvic floor variations separately, then practice them together. Notice the sensations as they work together. Be conscious of doing these exercises in a balanced manner. Overexertion of one group can decrease the optimal function of the other.

ABDOMINAL CORE BUILDER INSTRUCTIONS
VARIATION 1: LEG LIFT

1. Begin in Mountain Pose on the Earth (see page 221 for instructions).

2. Press the left leg and lower ribs into the earth, and press your left heel away from you.

3. Exhale and lift your right leg a few inches from the earth with a flexed right foot.

4. Pull your belly in and press your tailbone toward your heels.

5. Inhale and lower your right leg to the earth.

6. Practice steps 2-5 using the opposite side of your body. Raise the left leg while pressing the right leg and ribs into the earth. Match your breath to your movement.

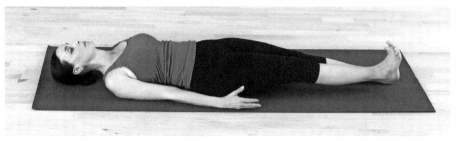

Variation 1: Leg Lift

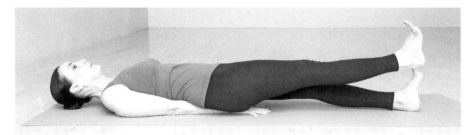

Variation 1: Leg Lift with hands under hips

7. Enjoy Variation 1: Leg Lift. Alternate lifting and lowering each leg for up to 3 to 5 repetitions.

8. For a greater challenge, practice holding the raised leg for 3 to 5 breaths before lowering on the inhale.

ADAPTATIONS TO VARIATION 1: LEG LIFT

- Place a blanket under your head if your head tilts back when you raise your leg.

- Practice with your hands under your hips if your back feels strained.

- Visualize lifting each leg alternately while in Mountain Pose on the Earth. Intentionally *do not allow* the leg to lift. Activate your core by pressing your ribs into the earth, pulling your belly in, contracting your thigh muscles, and pressing your heels away from you. Note that it is not necessary for your legs to lift off the earth to benefit from this core builder. The mind and body connection is powerful. Tune into the subtle sensations or actions in your body.

Yoga Moves Your Core

VARIATION 2: HEAD AND LEG LIFT

1. Begin in Mountain Pose on the Earth (see page 221 for instructions).

2. Place your hands behind your head with your elbows out to the sides.

3. Press the left leg and lower ribs into the earth, and press your left heel away from you.

4. Pull your belly in and press your tailbone toward your heels.

5. Exhale and lift your torso and right leg with flexed foot a few inches from the earth, gazing at your toes. Cradle your head in your hands, rather than pushing your head upward or straining your neck.

6. Inhale and lower your right leg and head down.

7. Practice lifting and lowering the left leg and torso in the same manner, matching breath to movement.

8. Enjoy Variation 2: Head and Leg Lift. Alternate practicing with each leg, for up to 3 repetitions on each side.

9. For a greater challenge, practice holding the raised leg for 3 to 5 breaths before lowering on the inhale.

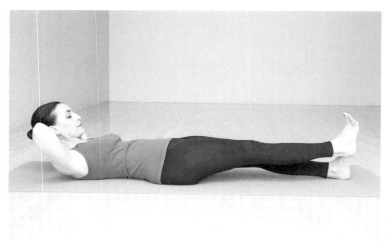

Variation 2:
Head and
Leg Lift

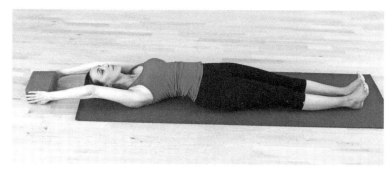

Variation 3: Arm Lift with block behind head

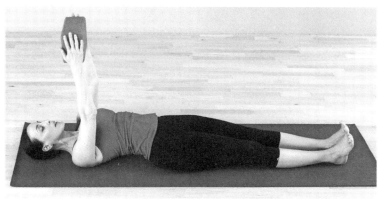

Variation 3: Arm Lift with block raised skyward

VARIATION 3: ARM LIFT

1. Begin in Mountain Pose on the Earth (see page 221 for instructions).

2. Place a block between your hands and press your palms into the short sides of the block.

3. Lift straight arms behind you and toward the earth.

4. Press your legs and lower ribs into the earth, pull your belly in, and press your tailbone toward your heels. Press your heels away from you.

5. Remain in this posture for 3 breaths.

6. Inhale and lift your arms skyward as you press your hands into the block.

7. Exhale and lower your arms behind you again. Be careful not to arch your back.

8. Enjoy Variation 3: Arm Lift for 3 to 5 repetitions, raising and lowering your arms to match your breath to your movements.

Yoga Moves Your Core

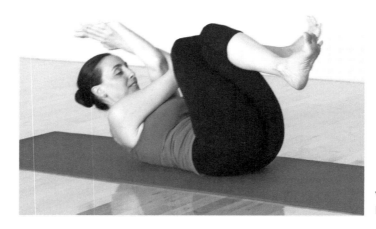

Variation 4:
Eagle Pose Curl

VARIATION 4: EAGLE POSE CURL

1. Begin in Bridge Prep Pose (see page 137 for instructions).

2. Cross your right elbow under your left elbow. Move your forearms toward each other. Your hands may or may not be able to grasp each other. This is called "Eagle" arms.

3. Cross your right leg over your left leg and hug your thighs and shins together.

4. Draw your belly in and lower your chin toward your chest.

5. Exhale, curl up, and draw your elbows and knees toward each other.

6. Inhale and return your head and feet to the earth, while maintaining "Eagle" arms.

7. Repeat instructions with arms and legs in these positions for 3 to 5 times, matching breath with movement.

8. Practice Variation 4: Eagle Pose Curl using the opposite side of your body. Cross the left elbow under the right elbow, and the left leg over the right leg. Repeat the curl 3 to 5 times on this side.

9. Enjoy Variation 4: Eagle Pose Curl, doing an equal number of curls on each side.

10. For a greater challenge, practice by gradually increasing the number of curls for up to 10 times on each side.

VARIATION 5: BUTTERFLY CORE BUILDER

1. Begin in Bridge Prep Pose (see page 137 for instructions).

2. Press the soles of your feet together. Open your knees to each side and down toward the earth in "butterfly" position. Place your hands stacked behind your head with your elbows out to the sides.

3. Exhale and curl up while pulling your knees toward each other. Gaze forward toward your toes. Cradle your head in your hands rather than pushing your head upward or straining your neck.

4. Inhale and lower your head and feet back to the earth, opening legs in "butterfly" position.

5. Enjoy Variation 5: Butterfly Core Builder for 3 to 5 repetitions.

ADAPTATIONS TO VARIATION 5: BUTTERFLY CORE BUILDER

- Practice with raised "butterfly" legs and feet. Lift your knees over your hips, with your feet together and raised from the earth, keeping your knees open in "butterfly" position. Cradle your head in your hands and curl up toward your "butterfly" legs as you exhale. Inhale, lower your head and keep legs raised. After the repetitions are completed, return feet to the earth with legs still in "butterfly" position. Relax for a few breaths.

- Practice with arms as shown in Variation 4: Eagle Pose Curl.

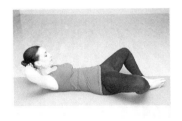

Variation 5: Butterfly Core Builder

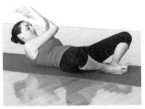

Variation 5: Butterfly Core Builder with "eagle" arms

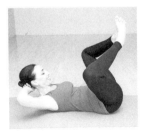

Variation 5: Butterfly Core Builder with raised "butterfly" legs

Yoga Moves Your Core

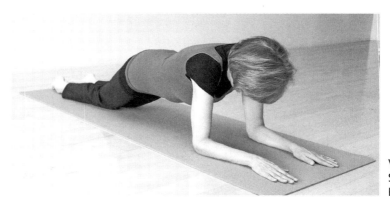

Variation 6: Sphinx Core Builder

VARIATION 6: SPHINX CORE BUILDER

1. Begin in Sphinx Pose (see page 266 for instructions). Your toes may be curled under or flat against the earth.

2. Pull your belly in and up.

3. Press your forearms and hands into the earth.

4. Tuck your chin to your chest.

5. Exhale, lift your hips off the earth, and curl your spine as in Cat Pose. Gaze at your belly.

6. Inhale and release your hips to the earth.

7. Enjoy Variation 6: Sphinx Core Builder for 3 to 5 repetitions. Cycle between contracting and releasing your muscles as you rock and roll with your breath.

ADAPTATION TO VARIATION 6: SPHINX CORE BUILDER

- Practice Plank Pose or Knee Plank Pose

PELVIC FLOOR CORE BUILDER INSTRUCTIONS

Many think of Kegel exercises when discussing the pelvic floor. However, Kegel exercises by themselves often lead to misunderstood instructions for proper pelvic floor toning. Too often, people clench their buttocks when they believe they are activating their pelvic floor muscles. This can be counterproductive. In addition, learning to release is equally important as learning to activate the proper muscles for a supportive pelvic floor.

Examples of symptoms for weak pelvic floor muscles include stress incontinence and pelvic organ prolapse, while symptoms of tight pelvic floor muscles include pelvic pain, urinary and bowel urgency, urinary frequency, constipation, irritable bowel syndrome, low back pain, and pain with intercourse. For symptoms of both under and over toned muscles, first address the symptoms of excessively toned muscles. If you are experiencing any of these symptoms, please consult with your physician.

AWARENESS OF PELVIC FLOOR MUSCLES

These practices bring awareness to the subtle sensations and inner workings of the pelvic floor. Begin these awareness practices in Bridge Prep Pose (see page 137 for instructions).

1. Find a neutral pelvis:

   a. Gently rock your hips backward and forward several times, alternating between arching and flattening your back to the earth.

   b. Find the midway point between a pelvic tilt forward and backward to find your neutral pelvis.

2. Find your most commonly used pelvic floor muscles:

   a. Contract and release the muscles used to halt urination.

   b. Contract and release the muscles used to halt passing gas.

   c. Contract and release both these muscle groups simultaneously. Avoid clenching the buttocks.

3. Release your pelvic floor muscles through breath and visualization:

   a. Begin in a relaxing pose such as Relaxation Pose (p 238) with a bolster under your knees, or Restorative Butterfly Pose (p 245).

   b. Inhale and visualize the pelvic floor widening and expanding.

   c. Exhale and visualize the muscles and the skin softening and relaxing.

   d. Repeat this visualization practice. Inhale a sense of spaciousness into the pelvic floor area, and exhale a sense of effortlessly releasing the skin and muscles. Let gravity do the work for you.

Yoga Moves Your Core

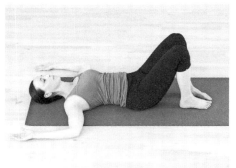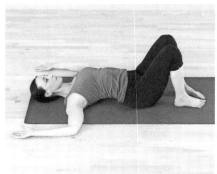

Variation 1: Pelvic Tilt Backward   Variation 1: Pelvic Tilt Forward

VARIATION 1: PELVIC TILT

1. Begin in Bridge Pose (see page 137 for instructions).

2. Exhale while tilting the top of the pelvis toward the earth and backward, so that there is no space between the earth and the back of your waist. The pubic bone curls upward. Contract your pelvic floor muscles for 1 to 3 counts in this position.

3. Inhale while tilting the top of your pelvis away from the earth and forward, so that there is space between the back of your waist and the earth. The pubic bone tips down and toward the earth. Release your pelvic floor muscles for 1 to 3 counts.

4. Enjoy Variation 1: Pelvic Tilt for 3 to 5 repetitions. Cycle between contracting and releasing pelvic floor muscles as you rock and roll with our breath.

5. As your practice becomes stronger, gradually increase the muscle contraction time for up to 10 counts, then releasing for up to 10 counts. You may practice this cycle for up to 10 repetitions.

VARIATION 2: PELVIC FLOOR CRUNCH

1. Begin in Bridge Prep Pose (see page 137 for instructions).

2. Cradle your head with your hands for support.

3. Exhale and lift your supported head at the same time as you tighten the pelvic floor muscles. Feel how your abdomen and pelvic floor tone as your lower back presses into the earth.

4. Inhale and return your head to the earth as you release your abdominal and pelvic floor muscles.

5. Enjoy Variation 2: Pelvic Floor Crunch for 1 to 3 repetitions.

6. For a greater challenge, hold the Pelvic Floor Crunch for up to 10 counts on each repetition.

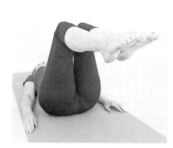
Variation 3: Toe Dip with shins parallel to earth and legs raised

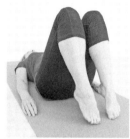
Variation 3: Toe Dip with toes touching earth

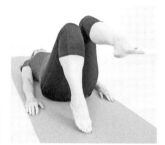
Variation 3: Toe Dip alternating feet

VARIATION 3: TOE DIP

1. Begin in Bridge Prep Pose (see page 137 for instructions).

2. Place your hands, palms to the earth, under your hips OR by your sides.

3. Exhale and lift both legs so that you knees are over your hips and the shins are parallel to the earth. Contract your pelvic floor muscles and pull your belly in and up.

4. Inhale, lower your toes to the earth, and release your pelvic floor muscles.

5. Enjoy Variation 3: Toe Dip for 3 to 5 repetitions, lifting and lowering your legs, matching breath to movement.

6. For a greater challenge, place your hands on top of your hip bones and maintain stationery hips.

ADAPTATION TO VARIATION 3: TOE DIP

• With knees raised over hips, practice alternating lowering and lifting one foot at a time.

Yoga Moves Your Core

VARIATION 4: MOUNTAIN POSE PELVIC EXERCISE

1. Begin in Mountain Pose standing (see page 220 for instructions).

2. Exhale, press down on the center of your heels, energetically hugging them together to tone your pelvic floor. Note that your leg muscles also engage with this hugging action when applying resistance between heels and the mat. Be careful not to lock your knees. Instead, bend them slightly.

3. Inhale and press your heels down and away from each other and release your pelvic floor.

4. Enjoy Variation 4: Mountain Pose Pelvic Exercise for 3 to 5 repetitions, alternately hugging your heels together to tighten your muscles and pressing them away from each other to release them.

5. Practice this variation at any time such as while standing in a crowd or in line at the store.

VARIATION 5: GODDESS POSE PELVIC EXERCISE

1. Begin in Goddess Pose in a Chair (see page 187 for instructions).

2. Exhale and energetically hug your heels toward each other without moving your feet. At the same time, tighten your pelvic floor muscles. Feel the sensation of your pelvic floor muscles engaged.

3. Inhale and release the muscle activation of the heels and pelvic floor.

4. Enjoy Variation 5: Goddess Pose Pelvic Excercise for 3 to 5 repetitions, alternating between contracting and releasing the pelvic floor muscles, matching breath to the movement.

5. For a greater challenge, practice in Goddess Pose standing.

VARIATION 6: CHAIR POSE PELVIC EXCERCISE

1. Begin in Mountain Pose in a Chair (see page 222 for instructions).

2. Place a yoga block between your thighs. Your hands may be on your thighs, OR your arms may be straight in front of you.

3. Hug the block between your thighs and tighten your pelvic floor muscles.

4. Exhale, lean forward, and rise into Chair Pose (see page 150 for instructions).

5. Hold Chair Pose for 1 to 3 breaths.

6. Inhale and slowly lower your buttocks to the chair and release the pelvic floor muscles.

7. Enjoy Variation 6: Chair Pose Pelvic Exercise, repeating instructions 1 to 3 times.

ADAPTATIONS TO VARIATION 6: CHAIR POSE PELVIC EXCERCISE

- Visualize lifting from the chair without your buttocks rising from the seat.

- Practice beginning in Chair Pose at the wall or freestanding Chair Pose.

- Practice Chair to Mountain Pose. From Chair Pose, exhale, press down through your feet, and rise to Mountain Pose for a Complete Yoga Breath. Continue to hug the block between your thighs. Inhale and return to Chair Pose for 1 to 3 breaths, before returning to your seat.

Yoga Moves Your Core

VARIATION 7: KEGEL EXERCISE

1. Begin in Mountain Pose, Mountain Pose in a Chair, OR Bridge Prep Pose (see pages 220, 222, OR 137, respectively, for instructions).

2. Isolate the muscles you use to halt urination.

3. Tighten these muscles for a count of 3.

4. Release these muscles for a count of 3.

5. Enjoy Variation 7: Kegel Exercises for 3 to 5 repetitions, tightening and releasing as you match breath to movement.

6. As your practice becomes stronger, gradually increase the holding time for up to 10 counts, then releasing for up to 10 counts before beginning the cycle again. You may practice this cycle for up to 10 repetitions.

 ### YOGA POSES TO MOVE YOUR ABDOMINAL CORE

See the "Index" to reference a few of these sample poses to warm up, tune up, and loosen up your core: Boat; Plank; Scale; Spinal Balance; and Stick.

 ### YOGA POSES TO MOVE YOUR PELVIC FLOOR

Postural alignment while seated, standing, or in yoga poses is fundamental for optimal pelvic floor tone. Choosing which postures to practice, and your approach to each posture, depends upon whether you are looking to strengthen your muscles or release tight pelvic floor muscles. See the "Index" to reference these sample poses to warm up, tune up, and loosen up your pelvic floor. Poses such as Butterfly; Happy Baby; Triangle; and Yoga Squat with a blanket supporting your heels, can be helpful for stretching a tight pelvic floor. Also, try some deeply relaxing poses such as Relaxation with a bolster under your knees, OR Restorative Butterfly, to release the pelvic floor muscles. Poses such as Boat with a block; Pelvic Tilts; and Plank can be helpful for strengthening the pelvic floor.

Yoga Moves Your Sides

PRIMARY BENEFITS

▨ Improves breathing

▨ Lengthens sides of body and opens rib cage

▨ Strengthens core

▨ Reduces effects of scoliosis

PRECAUTIONS

▨ Neck, shoulder, rib, or spinal condition, injury, or pain

PROPS

▨ Yoga mat

▨ Wall

▨ Chair

▨ Bolster

The sides of the body often compress during daily routines. While postural side bends are practiced asymmetrically, they bring symmetry and balance into your body.

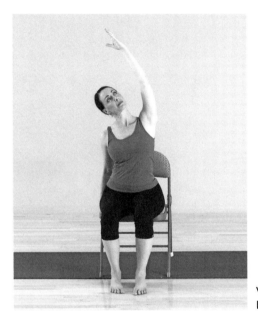

Variation 1: Side Bend in a Chair

INSTRUCTIONS
VARIATION 1: SIDE BEND IN A CHAIR

1. Begin in Mountain Pose in a Chair (see page 222 for instructions).

2. Place your right hand on the side of the chair.

3. Pull your belly in and up, lifting both sides of your waist to lengthen your torso.

4. Reach a straight left arm overhead.

5. Side bend to your right reaching toward two o'clock.

6. Press your right hand into the chair and your left hip into the chair to lengthen both sides of your body and deepen the stretch. An engaged belly will help too.

7. Gaze forward OR skyward.

8. Enjoy Variation 1: Side Bend in a Chair for 3 to 5 breaths.

9. Repeat the instructions above using the opposite of your body.

Yoga Moves Your Sides

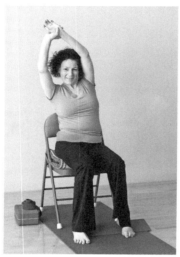

Variation 1: Side Bend in a Chair grasping wrist

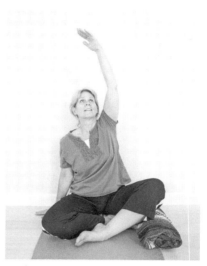

Variation 1: Side Bend in Easy Pose

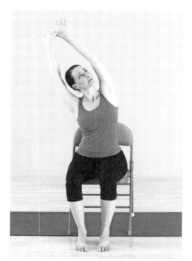

Variation 1: Side Bend in a Chair with thumbs interlaced

ADAPTATIONS TO VARIATION 1: SIDE BEND IN A CHAIR

- Use both hands overhead when you bend to each side.

- When bending toward the right, grasp your left wrist with your right hand and gently pull your left arm.

- Interlock your thumbs overhead and pull them away from each other as you lengthen your arms into a side bend.

- Practice beginning in Easy Pose (see page 175 for instructions).

VARIATION 2: STANDING SIDE BEND

1. Begin in Mountain Pose at the wall or in the middle of your mat (see page 220 for instructions).

2. Lift up long out of your waist as you reach both arms straight overhead.

3. Grasp your left wrist with your right hand and gently pull your left arm as you bend to the right.

4. Feel the stretch on the left side of your body while keeping the right side of your body long by drawing the right side of your belly in and up.

5. Press firmly into the earth with your left foot to enhance the stretch.

6. Enjoy Variation 2: Standing Side Bend for 3 to 5 breaths.

7. Repeat the instructions above using the opposite side of your body.

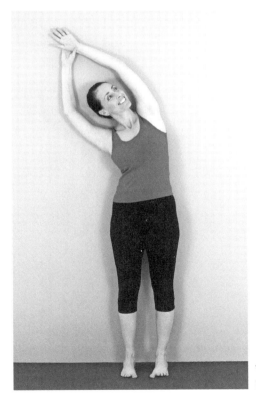

Variation 2:
Standing Side Bend

Yoga Moves Your Sides

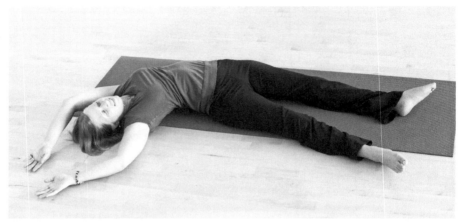

Variation 3: Side Bend on the earth

VARIATION 3: SIDE BEND ON THE EARTH

1. Begin in Mountain Pose on Earth (see page 221 for instructions).

2. Lift your arms overhead and to the earth.

3. Reach with both arms and legs toward the right into a side bend.

4. Feel the stretch on the left side of your body while keeping the right side of your body long.

5. Press your ribs and back of your legs into the earth.

6. Enjoy Variation 3: Side Bend on the Earth for 3 to 5 breaths.

7. Repeat the instructions above using the opposite side of your body.

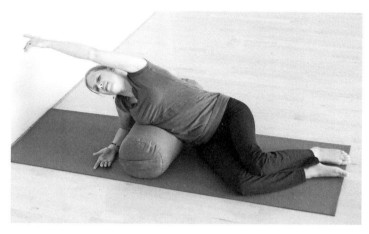

Variation 3: Side Bend on bolster

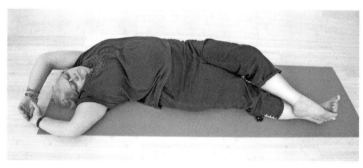

Variation 3: Side Bend on the Earth with crossed ankles

ADAPTATIONS TO VARIATION 3: SIDE BEND ON THE EARTH

- Grasp your left wrist with your right hand as you bend to the right.

- Cross your left ankle over your right shin and hug them together as you side bend to the right.

- Practice Side Bend on the Earth with a bolster. Place a bolster parallel to the top of your mat and lay on the bolster on your right side with your knees bent; lengthen your left arm over your ear.

YOGA POSES TO MOVE YOUR SIDES

See the "Index" to reference these sample poses to warm up, tune up, and loosen up your sides: Child's Pose Side Stretch Variation; Extended Side Angle; Half Moon; Pyramid; Spinal Twist Reclining; and Triangle.

Yoga Moves Your Hips, Legs, and Psoas

PRIMARY BENEFITS

■ Loosens hip joints

■ Massages spine

■ Lengthens psoas and hip flexors

■ Relaxes central nervous system (CNS)

■ Counters symptoms like foot drop

■ Increases awareness in the pelvis, hip joints, and legs

PRECAUTIONS

■ Leg, ankle, hip, or spinal condition, injury, or pain

■ Balance concerns

PROPS

■ Yoga mat

■ 1 or 2 chairs

■ Yoga block

Some people have naturally open hips and, therefore, hip openers in yoga feel blissful to them. For others who have tight hips, hip opening poses can be challenging but worth the effort to warm up, tune up, and loosen up your hips. The instructions here will prepare you for those challenging poses.

The psoas is a thick, long muscle connecting the upper and lower halves of your body. It extends from the lower back, through your pelvis, and attaches to your upper inner thigh bones. Conditioning the psoas muscle can impact your breath, nervous system, core strength, posture, how you walk and your sense of well-being.

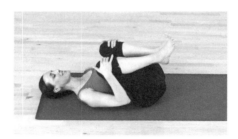

Variation 1: Juicy Hips
Spinal Massage

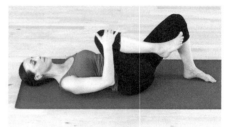

Variation 1: Juicy Hips
knee circles

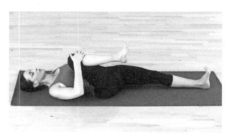

Variation 1: Juicy Hips
knee circles with one leg extended

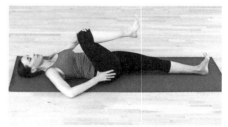

Variation 1: Juicy Hips with
finger in hip crease

INSTRUCTIONS
VARIATION 1: JUICY HIPS

1. Begin in Bridge Prep Pose (see page 137 for instructions).

2. Bring both knees to your chest placing your hands on your knees.

3. Roll forward and backward, and right to left several times, to massage the muscles around your spine.

4. Return to Bridge Prep Pose.

5. Raise your right knee and place your right hand on top of your knee or shin. Draw your right knee toward your chest and then away from you as your pelvis tilts backward and forward.

6. Return to Bridge Prep Pose.

7. Place your right hand on your right knee and lift it toward your chest, circling the leg and thigh in the hip joint 3 to 5 times. Begin with smaller circles and gradually make bigger circles to find your full range of motion within the hip socket. A common mistake is only circling the lower leg around the knee joint.

8. Return to Bridge Prep Pose.

9. Repeat the instructions above using the opposite leg.

ADAPTATIONS TO VARIATION 1: JUICY HIPS

- Extend your left leg straight down to the earth while holding a bent right knee. Press the left thigh into the earth with your left hand, while circling the right knee with your right hand.

- Circle both knees in opposite directions at the same time.

- Press your right thumb or fingers into the right hip crease to make space in your hip point, while circling your right knee with the left hand.

Yoga Moves Your Hips, Legs, and Psoas

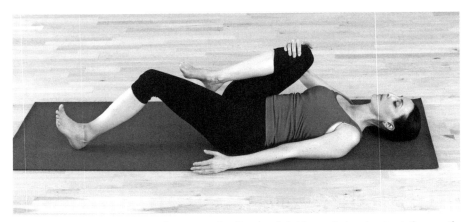

Variation 2: Psoas Release on the Earth, right knee into chest while gently
and slowly pressing the left heel away until the leg straightens

VARIATION 2: PSOAS RELEASE ON THE EARTH

1. Begin in Bridge Prep Pose (see page 137 for instructions).

2. Bring your right knee in toward you, with your right hand on top of your knee or shin.

3. Tilt your pelvis forward and backward until you find a neutral pelvis.

4. Gently press your left heel into the earth and away from you, as you slowly straighten your left leg. Maintain a neutral pelvis while straightening your left leg. If your pelvis shifts out of neutral, begin again.

5. Enjoy Variation 2: Psoas Release on the Earth for 3 to 5 breaths. Release your right leg and straighten it alongside the left leg.

6. Notice any difference between the two sides of your body.

7. Return to Bridge Prep Pose and find a neutral pelvis. Repeat instructions above using the opposite side of your body.

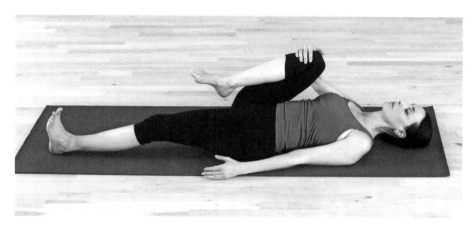

Variation 2: Psoas Release on the Earth

ADAPTATIONS TO VARIATION 2: PSOAS RELEASE ON THE EARTH

- When you bring your knee toward you in step 2, make circles with your right knee to open the hip joint before your straighten the left leg. After circling the knee, return to a neutral pelvis and continue with the remaining instructions, steps 3 through 7.

- Practice with a blanket under your head to maintain a neutral neck.

Yoga Moves Your Hips, Legs, and Psoas

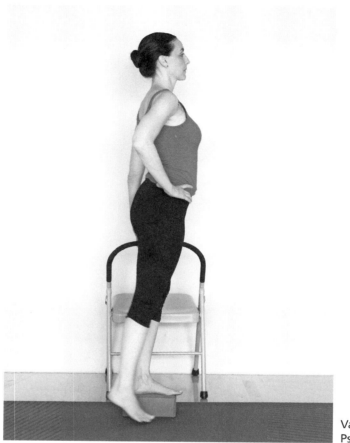

Variation 3:
Psoas Stretch

VARIATION 3: PSOAS STRETCH

1. Place a chair against the wall with the seat of the chair facing the wall.

2. Place a yoga block on the earth about six inches away from the back of the chair.

3. Stand next to the chair. Put your left hand on the back of the chair and step on the block with your left foot. This action will raise your right foot off of the earth.

4. Place your right hand on your hip.

5. Lengthen your upper body by lifting up through your heart and crown. Your spine will be long and tall.

6. Press your left foot into the block while activating your leg muscles. Place equal pressure onto the ball and heel.

7. Completely relax and let your right leg hang. Attune to your breath. Feel your right foot slowly lower toward the earth. It is a very subtle sensation.

8. Remain in Variation 3: Psoas Stretch for 5 to 10 breaths.

9. Repeat the instructions above using the opposite side of your body.

ADAPTATIONS TO VARIATION 3: PSOAS STRETCH

- Place a second chair next to your right side.

- Place a chair in front of you instead, with your left hand on your hip OR the wall, and your right hand on the chair.

- Practice without a chair, using just the wall for support.

Yoga Moves Your Hips, Legs, and Psoas

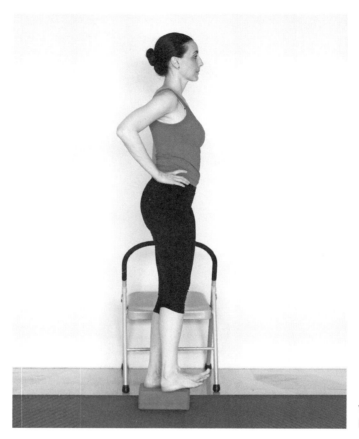

Variation 4:
Pendulum Swing

VARIATION 4: PENDULUM SWING

1. Follow instructions for Variation 3: Psoas Stretch, steps 1 through 6.

2. Flex your right foot and plug your right leg into your right hip socket. Your left standing leg is straight and energized. Be careful not to lock the left knee or lean into your left hip.

3. Energetically feel the connection between the right thigh bone and hip socket.

4. Swing the right leg forward and backward like a pendulum above the earth.

5. Enjoy Variation 4: Pendulum Swing 5 to 10 times with your breath.

6. Repeat the instructions above using the opposite side of your body.

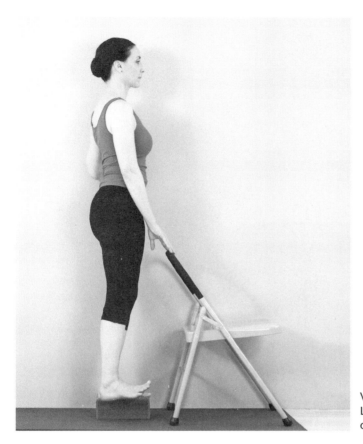

Variation 5: Hip Lift with alternate chair position

VARIATION 5: HIP LIFT

1. Follow instructions for Variation 3: Psoas Stretch, steps 1 through 6.

2. Flex your right foot and plug your right leg into your right hip socket. Your left standing leg is straight and energized. Be careful not to lock the left knee or lean into your left hip.

3. Energetically feel the connection between the right thigh bone and hip socket.

4. Lift and lower your right hip 5 to 10 times with your breath.

5. Increase the number of repetitions as you build strength.

6. Repeat the instructions above for Variation 5: Hip Lift, using the opposite side of your body.

Yoga Moves Your Hips, Legs, and Psoas

 ### YOGA POSES TO MOVE YOUR HIPS

See the "Index" to reference these sample poses to warm up, tune up, and loosen up your hips: #4, Butterfly; Crescent Warrior; Eagle; Firelog; Goddess; Half Lord of the Fishes; Happy Baby; Pigeon; Pyramid; Table Pose with Knee Circles; Triangle; and Warrior 2.

 ### YOGA POSES TO MOVE YOUR LEGS

See the "Index" to reference these sample poses to warm up, tune up, and loosen up your legs: Downward Facing Dog; Leg Stretch on the Back; Leg Stretch in a Chair; Legs Up The Wall; Mountain; Stick; Thigh Stretch on the Earth; Tree; Triangle; Wall Dog; Warrior 2; and Wide Angle Forward Fold.

 ### YOGA POSES TO MOVE YOUR PSOAS

See the "Index" to reference these poses to warm up, tune up, and loosen up your psoas: Bridge; Boat; Crescent Kneeling Lunge; Extended Side Angle; Pigeon; Thigh Stretch on the Earth; Tree.

Yoga Moves Your Feet

PRIMARY BENEFITS

■ Improves posture, alignment, and stability

■ Heightens awareness of soles

■ Builds strength and flexibility in ankles and feet

■ Improves health of fascia in feet

PRECAUTIONS

■ Foot or ankle condition, injury, or pain

PROPS

■ Yoga mat

■ Chair

■ Wall

■ Tennis ball

■ Yoga block

■ Lotion or oil

■ Socks

■ Toe separators

Feet represent our roots and foundation. We consider them primary to moving forward with confidence on this earth.

INSTRUCTIONS

Begin all variations in Mountain Pose in a Chair (see page 222 for instructions). Some variations may be modified to practice in a standing posture.

VARIATION 1: SOLE ENERGETICS

1. Inhale and sense your feet touching the earth.

2. Exhale and press the soles of your feet down. Specifically press evenly on the mounds of the big and little toes and the center of the heel. It is important to evenly distribute pressure throughout this triangle. Notice how the muscles of your legs activate.

3. Inhale and release.

4. Repeat Variation 1: Sole Energetics 3 to 5 times, matching your breath to the action.

VARIATION 2: ANKLE CIRCLES

1. Lift your right leg, OR interlace your fingers under your right thigh, OR use a strap to help lift your leg. You may keep your knee bent or extend your right leg straight.

2. Lengthen your upper body by lifting up through your heart and crown. Your spine will be long and tall.

3. Make circles with your right ankle both clockwise and counterclockwise.

4. Enjoy Variation 2: Ankle Circles 3 times in each direction.

5. Repeat the instruction above using the opposite side of your body.

Yoga Moves Your Feet

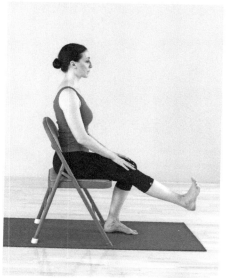 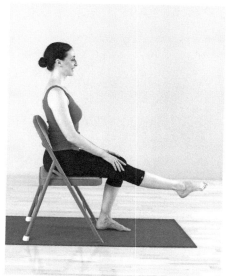

Variation 3: Flexed Foot   Variation 3: Pointed Foot

VARIATION 3: FLEX AND POINT

1. Lift your right leg, OR interlace your fingers under your right thigh, OR use a strap to help lift your leg. You may keep your knee bent or extend your leg straight.

2. Lengthen your upper body by lifting up through your heart and crown. Your spine will be long and tall.

3. Inhale and flex your right foot, drawing you toes toward you and pressing your heel away. Spread your toes. Feel your calf tone and the bottom of your foot lengthen.

4. Exhale and point your right toes. Feel the stretch along the front of the your right leg and the top of your foot.

5. Enjoy Variation 3: Flex and Point, alternating flexing and pointing your foot 3 to 5 times.

6. Repeat the instructions above using the opposite side of your body.

VARIATION 4: "FLOINT"

A "floint" is a combination of a pointed foot and a flexed foot, with your toes pointing toward you.

1. Lift your right leg, OR interlace your fingers under your right thigh, OR use a strap to help lift your leg. You may keep your knee bent or extend your leg straight.

2. Lengthen your upper body by lifting up through your heart and crown. Your spine will be long and tall.

3. Point your right foot.

4. Hold the foot steady. Flex only your right toes toward you, while pressing the big toe mound away from you.

5. Enjoy Variation 4: "Floint" for 3 to 5 breaths.

6. Repeat the instructions above using the opposite side of your body.

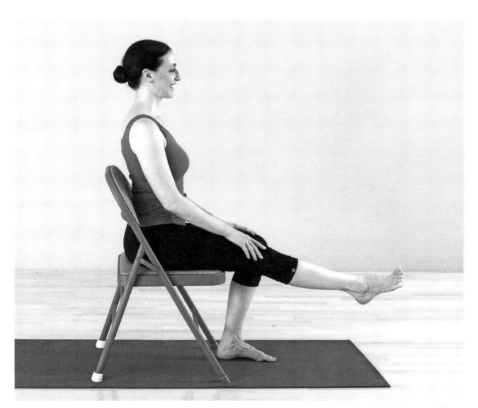

Variation 4: "Floint"

Yoga Moves Your Feet

I find I am able to do things that I didn't think I could do. I will never forget the first time, when we were standing, and you asked us to raise the toes on our right foot. I was unable to do that. However, the next time you asked, I was able to lift my toes! I was so excited! Seems like a small thing, but it was no small task for me.

JODI, YOGA MOVES STUDENT

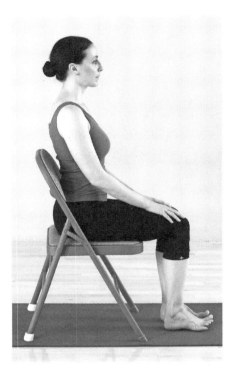

Variation 5: Toe Lift

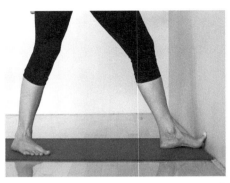

Variation 5: Toe Lift at the wall

VARIATION 5: TOE LIFT

1. Inhale and lift your toes. Spread your toes so that there is space between each toe.

2. Press evenly on the heels and balls of your feet.

3. Exhale and lower your toes, keeping them active.

4. Enjoy Variation 5: Toe Lift for 3 to 5 repetitions.

ADAPTATION TO VARIATION 5: TOE LIFT

• Sit or stand in front of a wall. Using one foot at a time, place your heel on the earth and your toes on the wall. Drag your toes down the wall until the ball of your foot is on the earth while your toes are still on the wall.

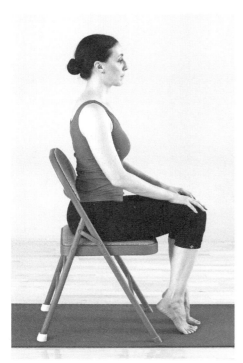
Variation 6: Heel Lift seated

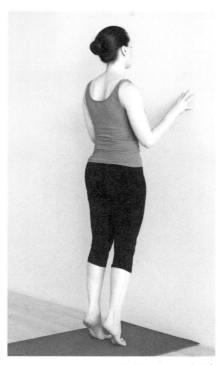
Variation 6: Heel Lift
standing at wall

VARIATION 6: HEEL LIFT

1. Inhale and lift your right heel straight up, pressing down evenly across the ball of your foot. Be careful not to roll toward the outside of your right foot.

2. Exhale and lower your right heel down maintaining parallel feet.

3. Repeat Steps 1 and 2 lifting your left heel.

4. Repeat and lift both heels at the same time.

5. Enjoy Variation 6: Heel Lift series for 3 to 5 repetitions.

ADAPTATIONS TO VARIATION 6: HEEL LIFT

• Practice standing at a wall. Be very cautious not to roll to the outside of your feet.

• Press a block between your thighs, shins, or ankles, and practice Heel Lift, seated or standing.

Yoga Moves Your Feet

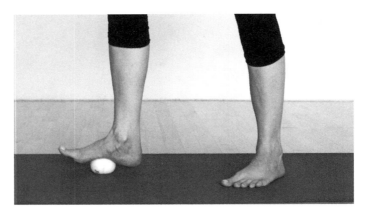

Variation 7: Pressure Point Foot Massage

VARIATION 7: PRESSURE POINT FOOT MASSAGE

1. While seated or standing, place your right foot on top of a tennis ball, and roll it slowly across the bottom of your foot on a yoga mat.

2. Enjoy finding different pressure points on the sole of your foot, and apply gentle pressure at each point as tolerated.

3. Enjoy Variation 7: the Pressure Point Foot Massage for 3 to 5 breaths.

4. Repeat the instructions above using the left foot. You may wish to place the tennis ball in a large box with low sides to prevent it from rolling away.

VARIATION 8: YOGA HANDSHAKE

1. Begin in #4 Pose (see page 130 for instructions).

2. Flex your right foot.

3. Weave your left fingers together with your right toes. This may be uncomfortable at first. Initially try weaving 2 or 3 fingers and work toward weaving all fingers and toes, interlaced to their webbing.

4. With your fingers and toes interlaced, circle your right ankle 2 to 3 times.

5. Repeat Variation 8: Yoga Handshake using the opposite side of your body.

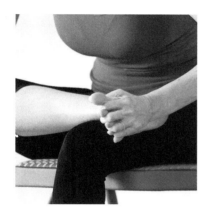

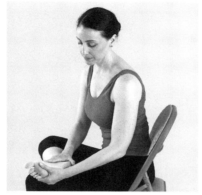

| Variation 8: Yoga Handshake | Variation 9: Foot Massage |

ADAPTATION TO VARIATION 8: YOGA HANDSHAKE

• Use products such as yoga toe separators throughout your day.

VARIATION 9: FOOT MASSAGE

1. Massage your feet daily at the end of your yoga practice, when you wake up, or before going to bed.

2. Use sesame oil, coconut oil or your favorite healing oil or cream while massaging your feet.

3. Massage the heel, the arch, the ball and toe pads of each foot. Massage each toe and between your toes.

4. Enjoy Variation 9: Foot massage for as long as you like.

5. Put socks or slippers over oiled feet. To avoid the risk of falling, do not walk on uncovered oiled feet.

Yoga Moves Your Feet

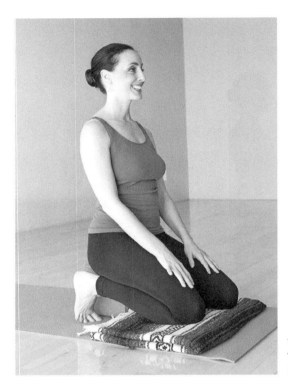

Variation 10:
Thunderbolt
Pose Foot Stretch

VARIATION 10: THUNDERBOLT POSE FOOT STRETCH

1. Begin in Thunderbolt Pose Variation of Hero Pose (see page 204 for instructions).

2. You may curl your toes under, OR lay them flat on the earth. Curled toes stretch the bottom of your feet while flat toes stretch the tops of your feet and ankles.

3. Note that each position works different foot muscles.

4. Enjoy Variation 10: Thunderbolt Pose Foot Stretch with your toes curled OR flat for 3 to 5 breaths. Work toward enjoying this pose longer as your foot muscle becomes accustomed to this stretch.

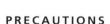 Yoga Moves Your Steps

PRIMARY BENEFITS

■ Stimulates bottom of feet and central nervous system (CNS)

■ Boosts mood and energy

■ Encourages rhythmic movement pattern

■ Contributes to heart and circulatory system health

■ Improves or maintains bone density

■ Simulates walking

PRECAUTIONS

■ Spine, knee, ankle, or foot condition, injury, or pain

PROPS

■ Yoga mat

■ Chair

■ Blanket

■ Cane, walker, scooter, or wheelchair

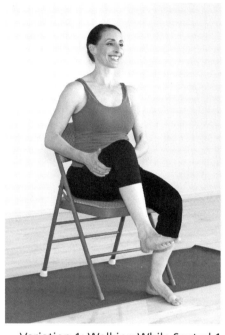
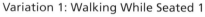

Variation 1: Walking While Seated 1   Variation 1: Walking While Seated 2

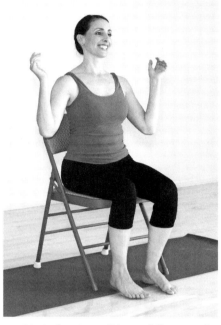

Walking represents stepping toward wellness and is one of the most natural ways to improve overall health. If we think about the complexity of movement and connections between body parts that go into our steps, we cannot help but be in awe. The previous Warm Up, Tune Up, Loosen Up sections give you a greater sense of the movement of different parts of your body. With Yoga Moves Your Steps, you can synthesize this knowledge while you walk. Use the variations below to invite awareness into your daily steps as you put your best foot forward.

INSTRUCTIONS
VARIATION 1: WALKING WHILE SEATED POSE

1. Begin in Mountain Pose in a Chair (see page 222 for instructions).

2. Lift up long through your spine, pull your belly in and lengthen your tailbone down.

3. Place your hands under your right thigh, inhale, and lift your right leg until the foot is between 3 to 12 inches off the floor.

Yoga Moves Your Steps

Walk as if you are kissing the Earth with your feet.

THÍCH NHAT HANH,
*PEACE IS EVERY STEP:
THE PATH OF MINDFULNESS
IN EVERYDAY LIFE*

4. Exhale and let go of your thigh, dropping your right foot to the earth with tender loving care. Concentrate on the sensations in your foot as your heel, ball, and toes touch the earth. You may change how lightly or heavily you drop your foot.

5. Repeat the instructions above lifting your left leg and dropping it.

6. Enjoy Variation 1: Walking While Seated. Alternate lifting and dropping each foot 8 to 10 times. Focus on finding a rhythm as you walk while seated.

ADAPTATIONS TO VARIATION 1: WALKING WHILE SEATED

- Experiment with allowing your heel or toe to touch down first.

- March while seated, lifting alternate legs without the assistance of your hands.

- Practice marching while standing, either in place, OR around the room. Consciously lift your knees high. This can help with foot drop.

VARIATION 2: MINDFUL WALKING MEDITATION

Mindful Walking Meditation is an alternative for those who cannot fathom sitting still to meditate, OR for those who wish to vary their meditation practice. By anchoring your mind with the rhythmic movement of your legs, you become aware of each step, and your mind becomes focused in the present moment on walking.

Practice Variation 2: Mindful Walking Meditation step by step, breath by breath, with acceptance, compassion, and loving kindness. Approach it with the curiosity of a beginner's mind, as though you have never walked before. If your mind wanders, simply guide it back to your steps and breath.

As you walk mindfully, you are not trying to change anything, although change may naturally occur. Some of my students tell me that their balance might feel off kilter when they so intently focus on their steps while walking. If you notice this too, stay safe, but know that as my students continue with the meditation, their balance often becomes stabilized.

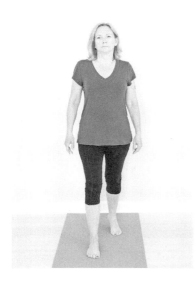

Variation 2:
Mindful Walking
Meditation

INSTRUCTIONS

1. Choose a path for Mindful Walking Meditation in your home, workplace, OR outdoors. You may walk in a circular pattern, back and forth, OR with no intended route.

2. Begin in Mountain Pose (see page 220 for instructions).

3. Shift your weight onto your left leg. Lift your right foot, swing it forward and place it down on the earth. Sense the heel, ball and toes as they sequentially touch down.

4. Shift your weight onto your right leg. Lift your left foot, swing it forward, and place it down on the earth. Sense the heel, ball and toes as they touch down.

5. Repeat, alternating sides, lifting, swinging, and placing each foot down. Your arms may remain by your side, or move freely with each step.

6. Notice any sensations, thoughts, reactions to your thoughts, or emotions that might arise. Merely label them as they are: sensations as sensations; thoughts as thoughts; reactions as reactions; and emotions as emotions. Acknowledge them, and let them pass, as though they were passing clouds in the sky. Return to your steps and your breath.

7. Enjoy Variation 2: Mindful Walking Meditation for 3 to 5 minutes, or up to 20 minutes.

Yoga Moves Your Steps

ADAPTATIONS TO VARIATION 2: MINDFUL WALKING MEDITATION

- Walk in place.

- Practice with bare feet or in shoes.

- Change your pace.

- Practice with a walker, cane, or next to a wall for assistance to help you safely ambulate.

- Practice Variation 2: Mindful Walking Meditation with a wheelchair or scooter. Be conscious of your breath, attune to your posture, arm and hand movements, and breathe as you move on this earth while meditating.

VARIATION 3: COMPASSIONATE STEPS

The objective of this exercise is to attune to how your body moves through space; to observe small segments of your steps, which when combined, propel you forward. Habit patterns for walking form during childhood and are impacted by life events and your environment. Long-term habits can lead to repetitive motion injuries, but some habits can be changed.

Compassionate Steps are made with great love for yourself, and without self-criticism or judgment. Be accepting and curious. Consider how you walk with the idea of preventing pain or imbalance, and acknowledge that there might be room for improvement. Ask yourself a few of the following questions while you walk:

Where is my gaze? Is it forward or down toward my feet? How are my head, spine and tailbone aligned? Am I leaning head first into my stroll? Does each foot lift off the earth as it swings forward? Do my knees bend or lock as I step? Does one foot or both feet turn out? Does my leg circle out to the side as I step? Do I step side to side with each foot? How long or wide is my stride? Do I feel a downward or upward energy as I walk? Do I tend to place weight on the inside or outside of my foot? Do my arms swing naturally and evenly?

Remember, these are potential questions to ask as you learn and accept your walking as it is. Once you begin noticing your subtle movements, you can make changes toward enhancing the way you walk as a gift to yourself. Please make a promise to yourself that you will not self-criticize while you practice Variation 3: Compassionate Steps.

INSTRUCTIONS

1. Choose a space for your Compassionate Steps, either a small limited space OR a walking path.

2. Begin strolling with your natural gait for 3 to 5 minutes.

3. Take note of your breath and intention.

4. As you stroll, refrain from labeling your gait as good or bad. Just walk and observe with loving kindness.

5. Consider observing one or two questions above while you stroll, without changing the way you are walking.

6. If your mind wanders, redirect it back to your steps, breath and intention.

7. After 3 to 5 minutes, experiment with changing one aspect of your movement pattern that you observed. For instance, if you notice your gaze is straight down to you toes, try to lift the gaze ahead of you as you stroll. If you notice that one foot drags, try slowing down your pace in order to lift the leg. Notice where the lift needs to originate. If you notice that a foot turns out, try reducing the turnout with each step by pointing your toes more forward. If you note that you tend to step side to side, try stepping forward with each leg instead. If you notice you walk with a downward energy, try reversing the energy upward by lifting up through your spine and crown as you stroll.

ADAPTATIONS TO VARIATION 3: COMPASSIONATE STEPS

- Walk in place.
- Practice with bare feet or in shoes.
- Change your pace.
- Practice with a walker or cane for assistance to help you safely ambulate.

CHAPTER 7

*"Yoga has changed my life. I try to do all of the poses.
Some are harder, and some are easier. There is something for everyone.
You can do more than you think if you just try!"*

MARGO, YOGA MOVES STUDENT

Adaptive Poses

Asanas

Get ready to engage in serious play with the following "Adaptive Poses". The practice of yoga is an inward journey and empowers you to take part in your own healing. The most important ingredients for practicing adaptive yoga are exploration, creativity, spontaneity, joy, and smiles.

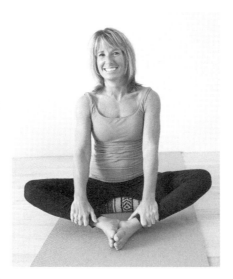

Poses, called *asanas* in Sanskrit, are postures or shapes formed with your body, and are consciously paired with your breath. Seventy-one traditional yoga poses, with many adaptations, are offered here in alphabetical order.

Instructions are given for how you approach and align your body in each pose. Instructions for asymetrical poses are given to practice on the right side first. For balanced practice, repeat the instructions on the left side of your body. The poses vary between physically challenging to deeply restorative. My Yoga Moves students inspired many of the adaptations presented here. I am confident you will create even more clever modifications. Be playful, the possibilities are endless.

To choose your poses for any given day, go inward. Ask yourself, "What does my body need today?" A positive attitude gently allows you to go beyond your comfort zone and surprise yourself with what you are capable of doing. You might begin with a Yoga Moves sequence, or you can be creative and combine yoga poses with selections from the "Warm Up, Tune Up and Loosen Up" chapter.

Take comfort knowing you are nurturing and fine-tuning your body, mind, and spirit. With adaptive yoga you can individualize the practice to your own needs and abilities. The most important yoga pose is your smile, and the most important words in your practice are, "Yes, I can!"

#4 Pose / Eye of the Needle

Sucirandhrasana

PRIMARY BENEFITS

■ Opens hips

■ Stretches inner thighs and outer hips

PRECAUTIONS

■ Low back, hip or knee condition, injury, or pain

PROPS

■ Yoga mat

■ Chair

■ Yoga strap

■ Yoga block

■ Wall

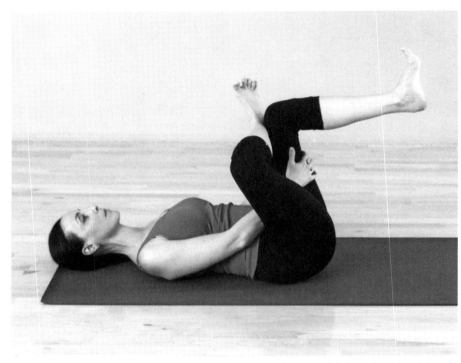

#4 Pose with hands behind thigh

POSE INSTRUCTIONS

1. Begin in Bridge Prep Pose (see page 137 for instructions).

2. Lift your right foot, rotate the knee outward, and rest your right ankle on your left thigh. You are making the number 4 with your legs.

3. Flex your right foot, spread your toes, and press through the ball of your big toe as though it were against a wall. This will protect your right knee.

4. Lift your left leg off the ground, flex your foot, and clasp your hands around the back of your left thigh, with your right hand going between your thighs. Gently pull the left thigh toward you as you press the right knee away from you.

5. Level your hips so you are not leaning to one side.

6. Enjoy #4 Pose for 3 to 5 breaths.

7. Practice the instructions above using the opposite side of your body.

ADAPTATIONS AND VARIATIONS

- In #4 Pose, keep your left foot on the earth if you feel a hip stretch.

- Clasp your hands around the front of your left shin instead of behind the left thigh. This intensifies the stretch in your hip.

- Practice #4 Pose with a strap by beginning in Bridge Prep Pose. Cross your right leg over your left thigh as in above instructions. Place a strap across the front of your thighs, and wrap it around them. Bring the ends of the strap between your thighs. Pull both ends of the strap to lift your left leg.

- Practice #4 Pose against a wall. Lie on your back with both of your feet on the wall and your knees bent at a 90 degree angle. Follow steps 2 through 7 above. Move your hips closer or further from the wall depending on your flexibility. You may press your left hand into the bottom of your right foot while your right hand or elbow is pressing the right thigh toward the wall.

- Practice #4 Pose seated with hands behind hips.

- Practice #4 Pose while seated in a chair. Follow instruction steps 2 and 3 above. Press your left hand into the bottom of your right foot while your right hand or elbow presses into right thigh or shin. You may fold forward over your bent right leg and place a block under your right hand on the earth.

- Practice Fire Log Pose (see page 180 for instructions).

- Practice Pigeon Pose (see page ??? for instructions).

I have learned that #4 Pose can help release the aching along my sciatic nerve This pose consistently offers me great relief by reducing or eliminating the 'white noise' levels of discomfort that I had been living with for many years.

CYNDI, YOGA MOVES STUDENT

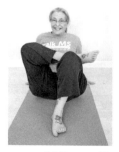

#4 Pose with
hands behind hips

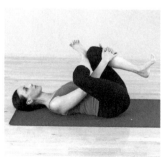

#4 Pose with
hands over shin

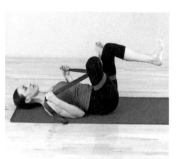

#4 Pose with
yoga strap

#4 Pose/Eye of the Needle

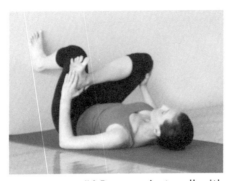

#4 Pose against wall with hand pressing into foot

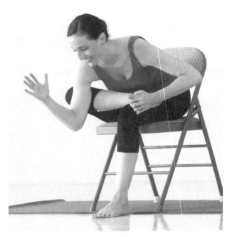

#4 Pose in chair, with elbow pressing into shin and hand on foot

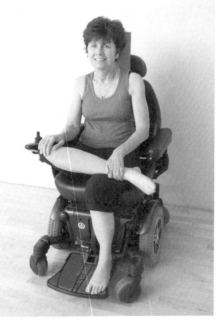

#4 Pose in chair

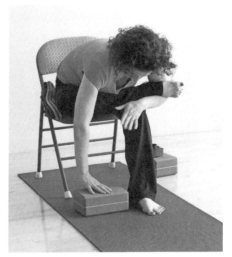

#4 Pose in chair with forward fold and block

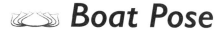 # Boat Pose

Navasana

PRIMARY BENEFITS

■ Builds core strength and stamina

■ Improves balance

PRECAUTIONS

■ Neck or spinal condition, injury, or pain

PROPS

■ Yoga mat

■ 1-2 chairs

■ Yoga block

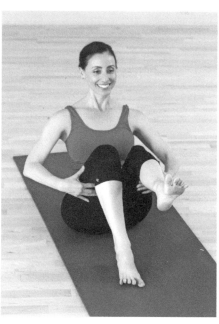

Boat Pose with hands behind thighs, one foot lifted, one on earth

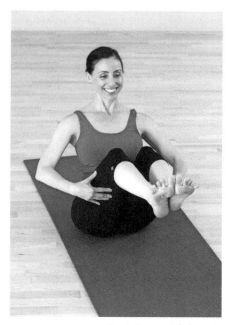

Boat Pose with hands behind thighs

POSE INSTRUCTIONS

1. Begin in Stick Pose (see page 276 for instructions).

2. Bend your knees and place your feet flat on the earth just in front of your hips.

3. Place your hands behind your thighs. Press your hands into your thighs and your thighs into your hands.

4. Lift your heart toward the sky and draw your shoulder blades together down your back.

5. Pull your belly in and up, and your tailbone down.

6. Lift your right foot a few inches from the earth on your exhale and lower the foot on the inhale. Repeat with the left foot. Repeat alternating feet a few times. You may wish to stop the pose at this point, OR continue.

Boat Pose

7. To find a place of balance and stability, begin to lean backward on your sitting bones. Experiment with moving your weight forward and back.

8. Continue pressing your hands and thighs against each other and lift both feet off the earth. Keep your feet lively and toes spread. Feel your belly engage.

9. Enjoy Boat Pose for 3 to 5 breaths.

ADAPTATIONS AND VARIATIONS

- If you experience lower back pain, draw your knees closer to you and lower your feet to the earth. If pain persists, discontinue the pose.

- Practice Boat Pose by leaning against a chair placed against a wall.

- Practice Boat Pose on two chairs, seated on one with your feet on another placed in front of you. You may press your hands into the chair seat as you lift your feet.

- Practice Boat Pose with a yoga block placed between your thighs.

- Practice Boat Pose while pressing your hands on the outside of your knees, and your knees pressing against your hands.

- Practice Boat Pose with your hands behind your hips on the earth, OR leaning back on your forearms.

- Vary the height that you raise your feet, either with bent knees, OR with straight legs.

- Release your hands while keeping your legs raised, and reach your arms forward, parallel to each other and to the earth, OR out to the side in a "T".

- From Boat Pose, open into a twist to your right side with arms in "T", one arm in front of you and one arm behind you. Practice the twist to the left side.

- When you are ready to build strength, extend both of your legs and lower them almost to the earth as you exhale. Then lift both legs to form a "V" shape with your body on the inhale. Continue raising and lowering for 3 breaths, increasing the duration as you build stamina.

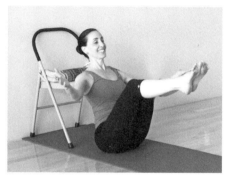

Boat Pose leaning on chair against the wall

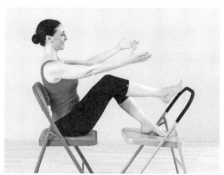

Boat Pose with two chairs, arms and one foot lifted

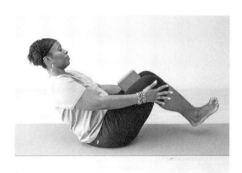

Boat Pose with block between thighs and hands pressing into knees

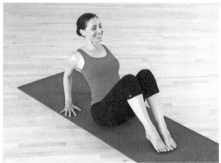

Boat Pose with hands behind hips

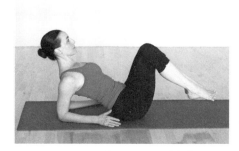

Boat Pose on forearms with feet up

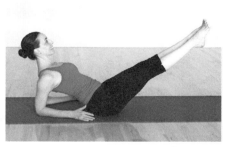

Boat Pose on forearms with legs fully extended

Boat Pose

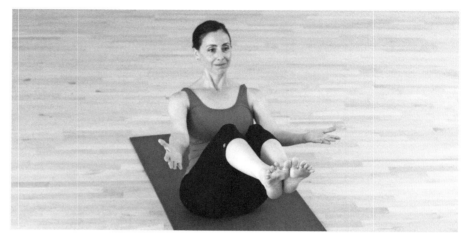

Boat Pose with arms and legs lifted

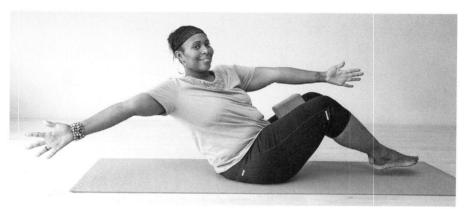

Boat Pose with twist and block between thighs

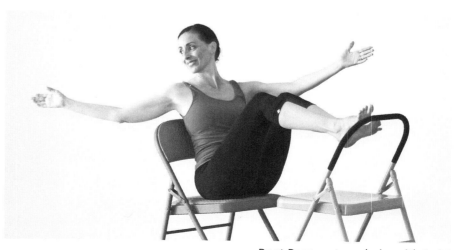

Boat Pose on two chairs with twist

Bridge Prep Pose and Bridge Pose

Setu Bandha Sarvangasana

PRIMARY BENEFITS

■ Opens shoulders and heart

■ Lengthens torso and thighs

■ Strengthens legs

■ Enhances mood

PRECAUTIONS

■ Neck, shoulder, knee, spine condition, injury, or pain

PROPS

■ Yoga mat

■ Yoga strap

■ Yoga block

■ Blanket

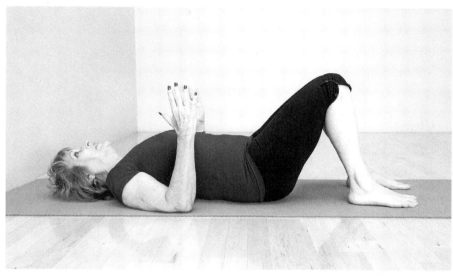

Bridge Prep Pose

BRIDGE PREP POSE INSTRUCTIONS

1. Begin on the earth on your back.

2. Bend your knees and place your heels under your knees, hip distance apart, and parallel to each other.

3. Place your arms into "robot" position with your elbows bent and pressing the upper arms into the mat. Your palms face each other.

BRIDGE POSE INSTRUCTIONS

1. Begin in Bridge Prep Pose (see above).

2. Press down through your feet.

3. Lift your hips, and move your heart toward your chin.

4. Continue to press down through your feet as you tone and firm your outer hips.

5. Enjoy Bridge Pose for 3 to 5 breaths.

Bridge Prep Pose and Bridge Pose

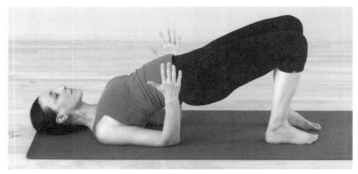

Bridge Pose with "robot" arms

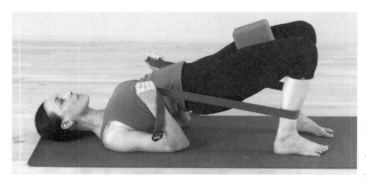

Bridge Pose with block between thighs and strap around shins

ADAPTATIONS AND VARIATIONS

- Place a yoga block between your thighs. As you press into the block to help you focus on your midline, you will activate your inner thighs and become more aware of your energetic center and core.

- Grasp a yoga strap gently in both hands, and place it around your shins for support.

- Place a block between your thighs and a strap looped around your thighs. You may need assistance with the strap.

- Place a blanket under your head so your head does not tilt back.

- Place a blanket under your upper back, with the edge of the blanket lining up with the top of your shoulders to support the natural curve in your spine.

- In lieu of "robot" arms, shrug your shoulders up to your ears and roll shoulders back to the earth. Interlace your fingers under your back.

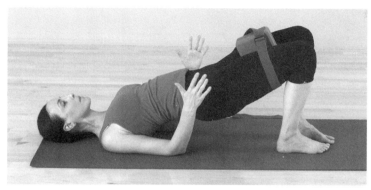

Bridge Pose with block between thighs and strap around thighs

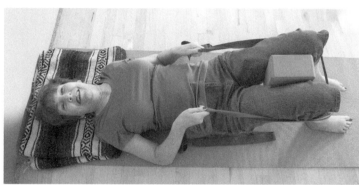

Bridge Pose with block, strap and blanket under head

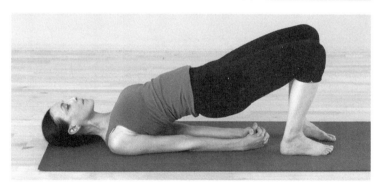

Bridge Pose with interlaced fingers

Butterfly Pose

Baddha Konasana

PRIMARY BENEFITS

■ Opens hips, inner thighs, and groin muscles

PRECAUTIONS

■ Spine, knee, and hip condition, injury, or pain

PROPS

■ Yoga mat

■ 1 to 2 chairs

■ Blankets

■ Yoga blocks

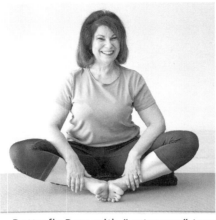

Butterfly Pose with "antennae" toes

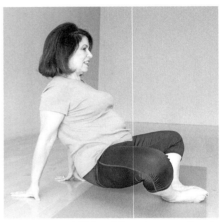

Lifting hips closer to heels

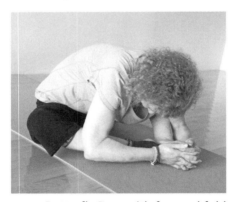

Butterfly Pose with forward fold

POSE INSTRUCTIONS

1. Begin in Easy Pose (see page 175 for instructions).

2. If your knees are high above your hips, sit on one or more blankets. This will also lessen a rounded back.

3. Widen your knees and press the soles of your feet together. Do not press down on your knee joints. Instead, allow them to open gradually.

4. Bring your heels and hips close together. Either hold your ankles and bring them close to your groin, OR place your fingers behind your hips and lift them forward toward your heels, OR both.

5. Press your feet together, especially the big toe mounds, and flex your toes ("antennae" of the butterfly).

6. Pull your ankles toward you to help lift your heart and spine.

7. Fold forward for an increased stretch.

8. Enjoy Butterfly Pose for 3 to 5 breaths.

9. Close your knees with your hands to exit the pose.

ADAPTATIONS AND VARIATIONS

- Place yoga blocks or blankets under your knees or hips for comfort.

- Practice Butterfly Pose on one chair with your toes down on the earth and heels together.

- Practice Butterfly Pose with two chairs, placing your hands on the top of the chair in front of you.

- Open your feet like a book, keeping the little toe sides together and your big toes opened apart.

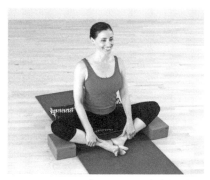

Butterfly Pose with blanket and blocks

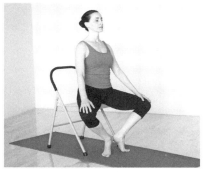

Frontal view of Butterfly Pose with one chair and toes down

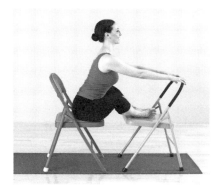

Butterfly Pose with two chairs and hands on top of second chair

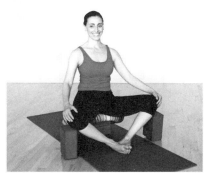

Butterfly Pose "throne" with blocks and blanket

Butterfly Pose

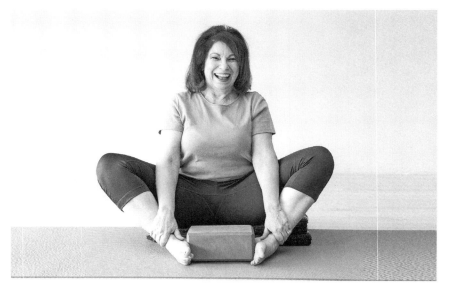

Butterfly Pose with block between feet

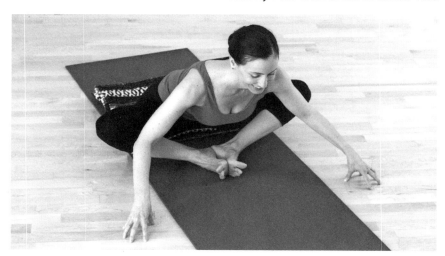

Butterfly Pose on blanket with forward fold

- Practice Butterfly Pose with a block between your feet in 3 consecutive positions going from narrowest to widest. Press your feet into the block for 3 to 5 breaths in each position. Finally, place the feet back together without the block and feel the difference in the height of your hips and knees.

- Press your hands against the inside of the thighs and your thighs into your hands with equal pressure to tone the inner thigh muscles.

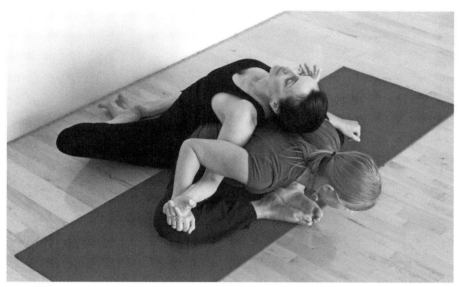

Butterfly Pose with a friend, position A

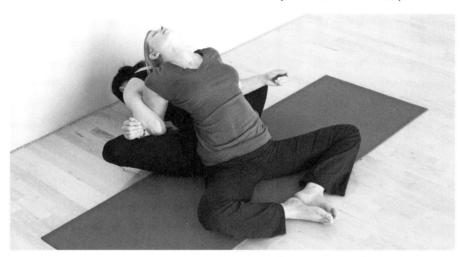

Butterfly Pose with a friend, position B

- Practice Butterfly Pose with a friend. Sit back to back and interlock elbows. Take turns folding forward (position A in photo) and backward (position B). Enjoy each fold for 3 to 5 breaths.
- Practice Restorative Butterfly Pose (see page 245 for instructions).

Camel Pose

Ustrasana

PRIMARY BENEFITS

■ Lengthens front of body, including thighs and hip flexors

■ Opens shoulders and

■ Increases energy and lifts one's mood

PRECAUTIONS

■ Lower back, shoulder or neck condition, injury, or pain

PROPS

■ Yoga mat

■ 1 to 2 chairs

■ Blankets

■ Bolster

■ Yoga blocks

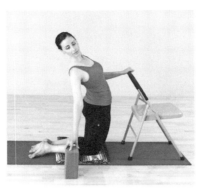

Camel Pose with one hand on block, one hand on chair

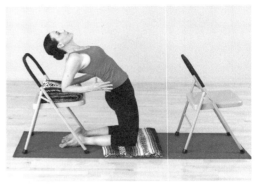

Camel Pose with two chairs and blankets

POSE INSTRUCTIONS

1. Place a chair on your mat.

2. Begin standing on your knees, cushioned by blankets, facing the back of the chair. Place a block by your right shin.

3. Place your hands on the back of the chair.

4. Place your knees hip distance apart. Stack your hips over your knees and your shoulders over your hips.

5. Press the tops of the toes into the mat, OR curl your toes under. Notice which foot position gives greater stability.

6. Lift up and out of your waist and draw your shoulder blades together onto your back.

7. Lift your belly in and up as you lengthen your tailbone down.

8. Begin a twist from your belly to reach your right hand back. Place your right hand on your right heel or the block. Your left hand may remain on the chair or on your left hip.

9. Keep your neck long without compressing it and open your heart skyward for this backbend.

10. Enjoy Camel Pose for 3 to 5 breaths.

11. With your head following last, return to standing on your knees by releasing your hand and placing both hands on the chair.

12. Practice the instructions above using the opposite side of your body.

ADAPTATIONS AND VARIATIONS

- Place a chair behind you and position your elbows on the seat of the chair OR a stack of blankets. You may place a chair in front of you for support exiting the pose.

- Place a block between your thighs to support your back.

- Practice Camel Pose with both hands on the back of a chair and a block between your thighs.

- Place a bolster behind your knees and reach both hands to the bolster.

- For traditional Camel Pose, follow the pose instructions placing both hands on heels at the same time.

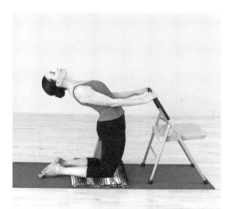

Camel Pose with chair,
block between thighs

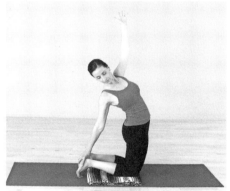

Camel Pose with one hand to
heel, one hand skyward

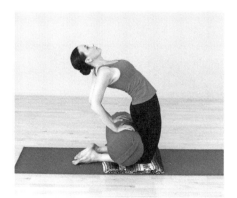

Camel Pose with
bolster behind knees

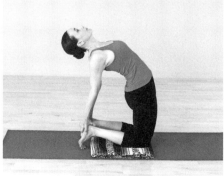

Camel Pose with both
hands on heels

Cat and Cow Poses

Marjari Bitilasana

PRIMARY BENEFITS

■ Warms up spine

■ Creates space between vertebrae

■ Brings awareness to upper and lower spine

PRECAUTIONS

■ Spine, neck, wrist, or knee condition, injury, or pain

PROPS

■ Yoga mat

■ Blanket

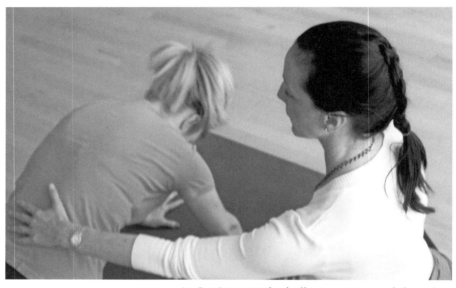

In Cat Pose, as the belly moves toward the spine, breathe into the lower back.

CAT POSE INSTRUCTIONS

1. Begin in Table Pose (see page 280 for instructions).

2. Exhale and initiate movement from the pelvis curving the spine up toward the sky like an angry cat. The tailbone curls down and the chin moves in toward the chest, as you draw your belly in toward your spine.

COW POSE INSTRUCTIONS

1. Return to Table Pose.

2. Inhale and initiate movement from the pelvis to reverse the curve of the cat into the arch of a cow's back.

3. Move your inner thighs back and wide as you lift your tailbone.

4. Draw your shoulder blades together on your back.

5. Your middle spine and belly curve down toward the earth like a complacent cow. The sitting bones and neck curl upwards.

6. Keep the front and back of the neck long.

COMBINED CAT COW POSE INSTRUCTIONS

1. Beginning in Table Pose, practice the Cat Pose and the Cow Pose, one following the other, repeatedly, in a wavelike motion.

2. Let your breath lead each movement, as the spine rounds and arches and the pelvis moves backward and forward.

3. Alternate the movement, from Cat Pose to Cow Pose, 3 to 5 times.

ADAPTATIONS AND VARIATIONS

- Place a folded blanket under your knees.
- Practice Cat and Cow Poses on forearms with elbows under your shoulders.
- Practice Cat and Cow Poses in a Chair (see page 148 for instructions).
- Practice Pelvic Tilt Pose (see page 224 for instructions).

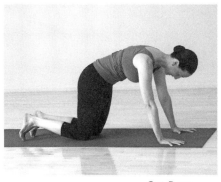

Cat Pose

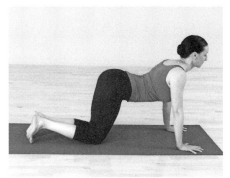

Cow Pose

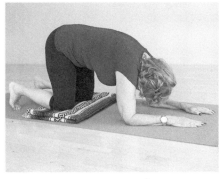

Cat Pose on forearms

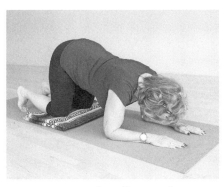

Cow Pose on forearms

Cat and Cow Poses in a Chair

Marjari Bitilasana Variation

PRIMARY BENEFITS

■ Warms up spine

■ Creates space between vertebrae

■ Brings awareness to upper and lower spine curvatures

PRECAUTIONS

■ Spinal or neck condition, injury, or pain

PROPS

■ Yoga mat

■ Chair

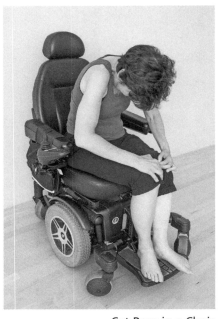
Cat Pose in a Chair

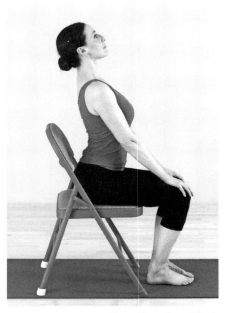
Cow Pose in a Chair

CAT POSE IN A CHAIR INSTRUCTIONS

1. Begin in Mountain Pose in a Chair (see page 222 for instructions).

2. Place your hands on your thighs or knees.

3. Exhale and initiate the movement from the pelvis while curving the spine back like an angry cat. The tailbone curls down and chin moves in toward your chest, as you draw your belly in toward your spine.

COW POSE IN A CHAIR INSTRUCTIONS

1. Return to Mountain Pose in a Chair.

2. Inhale and initiate the movement from the pelvis to reverse the curve of the cat into the arch of a cow's back.

3. Draw your shoulder blades together down your back

4. Your middle spine arches like a complacent cow. The sitting bones and neck curl back.

5. Keep the neck long and not compressed.

COMBINED CAT AND COW POSES INSTRUCTIONS

1. Begin in Mountain Pose in a Chair.

2. Practice the Cat Pose and the Cow Pose, one following the other, repeatedly, in a wavelike motion. Exhale in Cat Pose and inhale in Cow Pose.

3. Let your breath lead each movement. As the spine rounds and arches, the pelvis move forward and backward.

4. Alternate the movement, from Cat Pose to Cow Pose, 3 to 5 times.

ADAPTATIONS AND VARIATIONS

- Practice Cat and Cow Poses (see page 146 for instructions).
- Practice Inchworm Pose (see page 205 for instructions).
- Practice Pelvic Tilt Pose (see page 224 for instructions).

Chair Pose

Utkatasana Variation

PRIMARY BENEFITS

■ Strengthens thighs, calves, and ankles

■ Lengthens spine

PRECAUTIONS

■ Balance concerns

■ Knee or ankle condition, injury, or pain

PROPS

■ Yoga mat

■ Yoga blocks

■ Chair

■ Wall

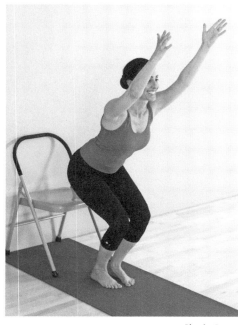

Chair Pose

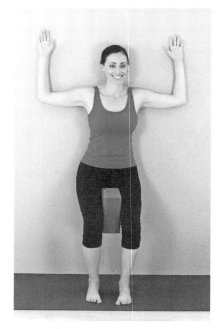

Chair Pose at wall with block between thighs and "cactus" arms

POSE INSTRUCTIONS

1. Place a chair with back against the wall.

2. Begin in Mountain Pose in a Chair (see page 222 for instructions).

3. Sit on the edge of the chair with your feet hip distance apart, and knees aligned with middle toes.

4. Lean forward on your sitting bones.

5. Raise your arms overhead, in line with your ears and press down through your feet. Draw your shoulder blades together on your back.

6. Draw your tailbone down toward the earth, and lift your belly in and up.

7. Rock back and forth creating momentum to lift your hips off the chair. The lift can be a millimeter or several inches but keep your knees bent.

8. Remain in Chair Pose, with your buttocks off the chair, for 3 to 5 breaths.

9. Slowly and gently lower your hips back down to the chair.

ADAPTATIONS AND VARIATIONS

- Place your hands on your thighs or hips.
- Place your arms shoulder height in front of you.
- Place a block between your thighs.
- Increase the time you remain in Chair Pose to increase strength.
- Practice Chair Pose at the wall:

  1. Begin standing in Mountain Pose (see page 220 for instructions) with your back against the wall. You may place a block between your thighs.
  2. Walk your feet about a foot forward.
  3. Press your spine into the wall as you lower down.
  4. Bend your knees so they line up with your middle toes.
  5. Place your arms in "cactus" against the wall with your elbows slightly below your shoulders.
  6. Place your hands on the wall behind your hips before exiting the pose.

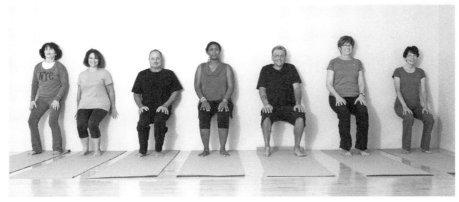

Chair Pose Chorus Line

Chair Pose

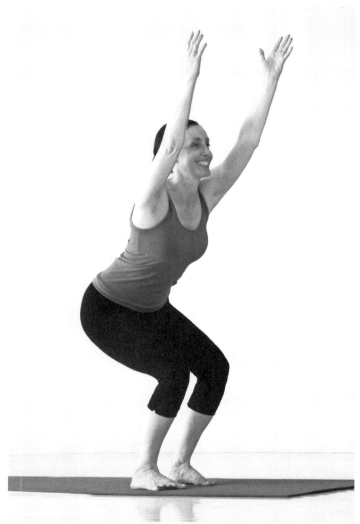

Freestanding
Chair Pose

- Practice freestanding Chair Pose:
    1. Begin in Mountain Pose (see page 220 for instructions) in the middle of your mat.
    2. Bend your knees deeply, aligning them over your middle toes.
    3. Raise your arms overhead in line with your ears.
    4. Keep your heart lifted, and draw your shoulder blades together on your back.
    5. Lengthen your tailbone down, and lift your belly in and up.

Child's Pose

Balasana

PRIMARY BENEFITS

- Calms and centers mind

- Releases tension in spine, shoulders, and hips

- Stretches spine, shoulders, hips, thighs, and ankles

- Provides a resting pose between more active poses

PRECAUTIONS

- Neck, shoulder, hip, knee, or ankle condition, injury, or pain

PROPS

- Yoga mat
- Yoga block
- Blankets
- Bolster
- Chairs

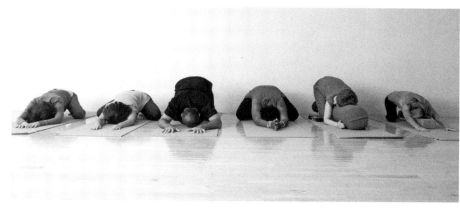

Child's Pose

POSE INSTRUCTIONS

1. Begin in Table Pose (see page 280 for instructions).

2. Touch your big toes together behind you and widen your knees a little more than hip distance apart. Adjust the width between your knees, wider or narrower, according to your comfort.

3. Sit back toward your heels. If your hips do not touch your heels, place blankets between your thighs and your calves until your hips rest comfortably on the blankets.

4. Walk your hands forward.

5. Rest your forehead on the mat, OR on a folded blanket, OR on a yoga block.

6. Allow the muscles of your spine and arms to relax.

7. Soften your belly with the natural in and out flow of your breath. Take this opportunity to breathe into the back of your body.

8. For a restorative pose, remain in Child's Pose for 1 to 3 minutes. If the pose is intended to be a resting pose between other yoga poses, enjoy Child's Pose for 3 to 5 breaths.

9. To come out of the pose, walk your hands back toward your knees and return to Table Pose.

Child's Pose

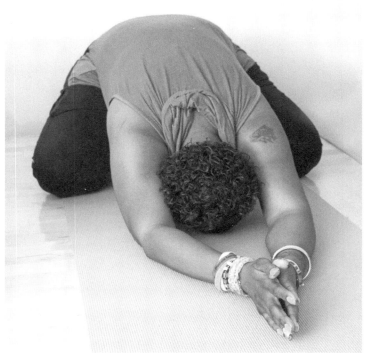

Child's Pose

ADAPTATIONS AND VARIATIONS

- Place a blanket under your ankles or feet for foot cramps.
- Place blankets under your forearms for shoulder comfort.
- Place a rolled washcloth behind your knees to lessen a pinching sensation.
- Bring your knees close together with the belly resting on the thighs.
- Place your arms behind you along your sides, with your palms facing skyward.
- Practice Active Child's Pose. Draw your belly in and up, and your tailbone down, to engage your core muscles.
- Practice Supported Child Pose. Place a bolster OR stacked blankets under your torso. You may turn your head to one side. If you do turn your head, make sure to spend equal time on each side.

- Practice Child's Pose Side Stretch. Walk your arms to the right and pull your left hip to the earth to lengthen the left side of your body and form a crescent shape. Breathe into the left side of your ribs for 3 to 5 breaths. Then walk your arms to the left and pull your right hip to the earth, breathing into the right side of your ribs. Return to center.

- Practice Child's Pose with two chairs facing each other. Begin seated on one chair, with knees wide. Lean forward and rest your arms on the facing chair. You may rest your head on stacked arms, blankets OR a block.

- Practice Puppy Pose (see page 234 for instructions).

One night, I was unable to find a comfortable sleeping position. I got out of bed and into a Child's Pose on the floor. I could feel everything shifting and relaxing inside my ribcage. My breathing came easier and my whole body eased up and relaxed. Quite simply, it felt as though this pose reset my whole body. I returned to bed for a restful sleep.

CYNDI, YOGA MOVES STUDENT

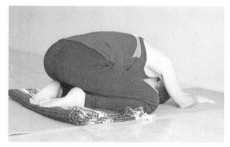

Child's Pose with blanket under ankles

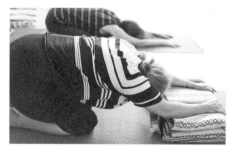

Child's Pose with blankets under forearms and hands

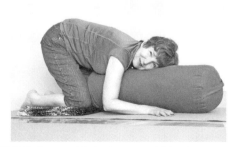

Child's Pose with bolster and blanket

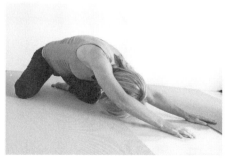

Child's Pose Side Stretch

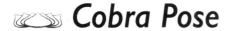 # Cobra Pose

Bhujangasana

PRIMARY BENEFITS

■ Opens shoulders and heart center

■ Lengthens front of body

■ Strengthens upper body

■ Stimulates digestive organs

PRECAUTIONS

■ Lower back, shoulder, or neck condition, injury, or pain.

■ Pregnancy

PROPS

■ Yoga mat

■ Yoga strap

■ Yoga block

■ Bolster

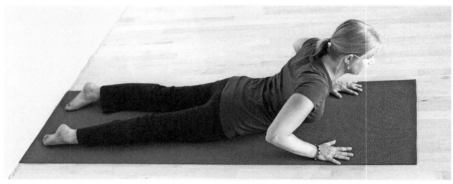

Cobra Pose

COBRA POSE INSTRUCTIONS

1. Begin on your belly.

2. Place your palms on the earth under your shoulders, with your elbows bent and hugging in toward your sides.

3. Point your toes straight back from your sitting bones. Spread and press them into the mat.

4. Draw your navel in and up as you lengthen your tailbone toward your heels.

5. Press the palms into the mat and energetically pull them back toward your hips.

6. In a fluid movement, lift your chest and shoulders off the mat, lengthen your torso, and draw your shoulder blades together onto your back.

7. Lengthen your neck and lift your head, while telescoping your heart forward and up.

8. Keep your gaze forward and your heart expanding.

9. Enjoy Cobra Pose for 3 to 5 breaths.

ADAPTATIONS AND VARIATIONS

• Widen your hands, press your fingertips down and lift your palms to make "spider" hands.

• Look over your right shoulder and roll it back; look over the left shoulder and roll it back. Alternate in a wavelike movement between shoulder rolls.

- Play with the width between your hands on the mat to find what produces the optimal shoulder opening for you.

- Rotate hands out to the side, OR inward to feel how that impacts your sense of having your shoulder blades together on the back.

- Place a block between your legs and have a friend wrap a strap around your calves to reduce any lower back pain, and to go into a deeper backbend.

- Place a rolled blanket or bolster under your chest.

- Practice Cobra Pose while standing facing a wall.

- Practice Cobra in a Chair at the Wall (see page 158 for instructions).

- Practice Locust Pose (see page 218 for instructions).

- Practice Sphinx Pose (see page 266 for instructions).

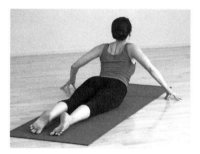

Cobra Pose with "spider" hands backview

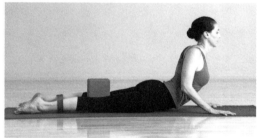

Cobra Pose with block and strap

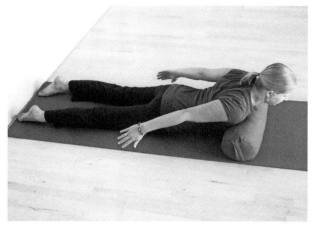

Cobra Pose with bolster

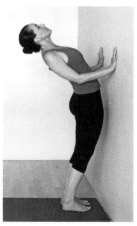

Cobra Pose at wall

Cobra Pose in a Chair at the Wall

Bhujangasana Variation

PRIMARY BENEFITS

■ Opens shoulders, heart center, and inner thighs

■ Lengthens front of body

■ Strengthens upper body

PRECAUTIONS

■ Wrist, neck, or shoulder condition, injury, or pain

PROPS

■ Yoga mat

■ Yoga blocks

■ Chair

■ Wall

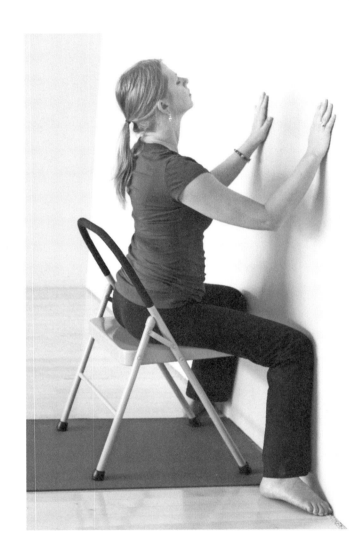

Cobra Pose in a Chair at the Wall

POSE INSTRUCTIONS

1. Begin in a chair facing the wall. Widen your knees and feet so that you are very close to the wall.

2. Place your feet under your knees with toes and knees pointing in the same direction.

3. Place your palms on the wall, shoulder height and shoulder width apart, with your fingers spread.

4. Draw your navel in and up, and lengthen tailbone down.

5. Lengthen the sides of your body as you press your palms into the wall.

6. Energetically draw your palms down and telescope your heart forward and up.

7. Draw your shoulder blades together on your back.

8. Keep the back of your neck long and your heart expanding.

9. Enjoy Cobra Pose in a Chair at the Wall for 3 to 5 breaths.

ADAPTATIONS AND VARIATIONS

- Rotate hands out to the side or inward to feel how that impacts your sense of having your shoulder blades together on the back.

- Practice Sphinx Pose in a chair at the wall (see page 267 for instructions).

Crescent Pose in a Chair

Virabhadrasana Variation

PRIMARY BENEFITS

■ Lengthens front of thighs and entire front of body

■ Opens shoulders and chest

■ Improves balance

PRECAUTIONS

■ Knee, ankle or hip condition, injury, or pain

PROPS

■ Yoga mat

■ Chair

■ Yoga blocks

■ Blanket

■ Yoga strap

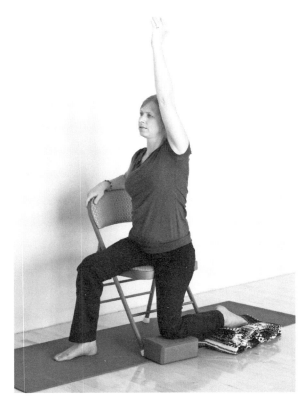

Crescent Pose in a Chair with arm raised, yoga block and blanket

POSE INSTRUCTIONS

1. Position yourself, sitting sideways in a chair with the right side of your body facing the back of the chair.
2. Place your right hand on the back of the chair for balance.
3. Place the front of your left knee and the top of your left foot on the mat, OR you may curl your left toes under. Avoid rolling your ankle in OR out.
4. Lift your belly in and up as you lengthen your tailbone down.
5. Position your shoulders over your hips.
6. Once you are in the pose, lengthen your left arm skyward, alongside your left ear. Gaze forward OR toward your raised hand.
7. Enjoy Crescent Pose in a Chair for 3 to 5 breaths.
8. Practice the instructions above using the opposite side of your body.

ADAPTATIONS AND VARIATIONS

- Use a block or a blanket to cushion knee or ankle.

- Move your entire right thigh onto the seat of the chair, and move your left hip and leg off the chair. Straighten your left leg behind you, curl your toes under and press through your back heel.

- Practice Crescent Pose in a Chair with a twist. Place both hands on the chair and twist to the right to face the wall.

- Reach both arms skyward in line with your ears.

- Practice Crescent Warrior Pose (see page 166 for instructions).

- Practice Thigh Stretch Pose on the Earth (see page 288 for instructions).

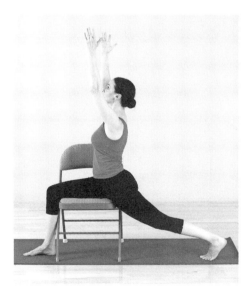

Crescent Pose in a Chair with both arms lifted, right thigh on chair and left leg straightened

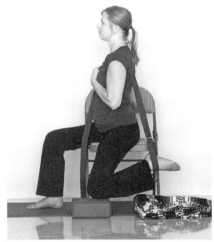

Crescent Pose in a Chair with yoga strap, block, and blanket

Crescent Kneeling Lunge Pose

Anjaneyasana

PRIMARY BENEFITS

- Lengthens front of thighs
- Strengthens legs
- Opens heart
- Improves balance

PRECAUTIONS

- Balance concerns
- Hip, knee, or ankle condition, injury, or pain

PROPS

- Yoga mat
- Yoga blocks
- Chair
- Wall
- Blanket

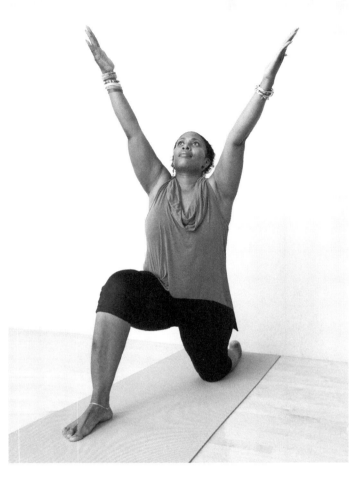

Crescent Kneeling Lunge Pose

POSE INSTRUCTIONS

1. Begin in Table Pose (see page 280 for instructions).

2. Bring your right foot forward between your hands, keeping your left knee on the earth.

3. Bend your right front knee beyond your ankle. Make sure the knee tracks over your middle toe.

4. Distribute weight in the left leg just above the kneecap. Do not place weight directly on the kneecap.

5. Curl your left toes under to activate the arch in your foot, OR maintain a straight ankle with the top of the left foot pressing into the earth. Avoid rolling your ankle in OR out.

6. Place your hands on top of your right thigh.

7. In a fluid movement, energetically hug your knees and feet toward each other, scoop your right hip down, pull your belly in, and press both hands into your right thigh to lift up and out of your waist.

8. Lift one or both of your arms overhead in line with your ears and draw your shoulder blades together on your back.

9. Lengthen your neck as you gaze skyward.

10. Enjoy the Crescent Kneeling Lunge Pose for 3 to 5 breaths.

11. Return to Table Pose.

12. Practice instructions above using the opposite side of your body.

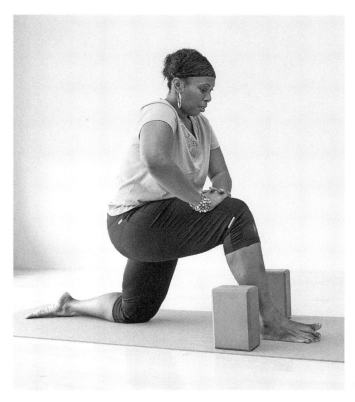

Crescent Kneeling
Lunge Pose prep
with hands on thigh

Crescent Kneeling Lunge Pose

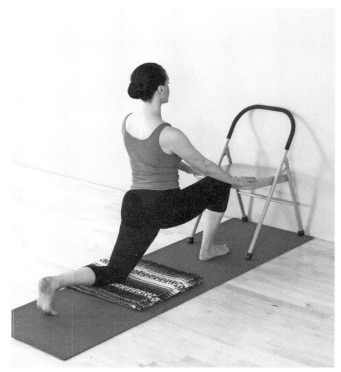

Crescent Kneeling
Lunge Pose with
chair against wall,
hands on chair seat

ADAPTATIONS AND VARIATIONS

- Use two yoga blocks, one under each hand, for increased height and balance.

- Practice Crescent Kneeling Lunge Pose with a blanket under your knee for padding.

- Practice Crescent Kneeling Lunge Pose with a chair. Place a chair against a wall and your front knee against the front of the chair seat. Raise one OR both arms overhead, OR cradle the back of your head with fingers interlaced, and lift your heart into a deeper backbend.

- Practice Crescent Pose in a Chair (see page 160 for instructions).

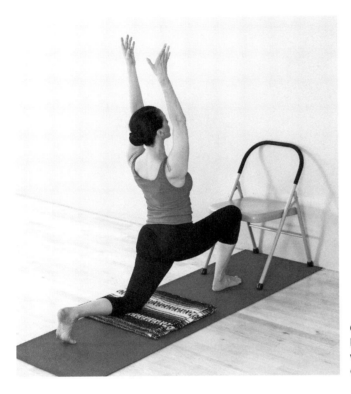

Crescent Kneeling
Lunge Pose at wall
with chair, arms
overhead

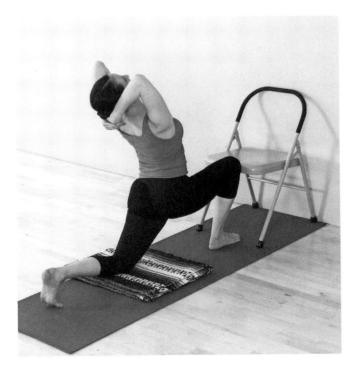

Crescent Kneeling
Lunge Pose at wall
with chair, hands
cradling head

Crescent Warrior Pose

Virabhadrasana

PRIMARY BENEFITS

■ Stretches thighs and groin

■ Strengthens legs

■ Opens heart

■ Improves balance

PRECAUTIONS

■ Balance concerns

■ Lower back, hip, knee, or ankle condition, injury, or pain

PROPS

■ Yoga mat

■ Yoga blocks

■ Chair

■ Wall

■ Blanket

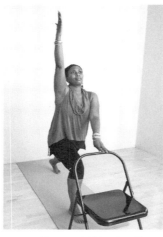

Crescent Warrior Pose with chair

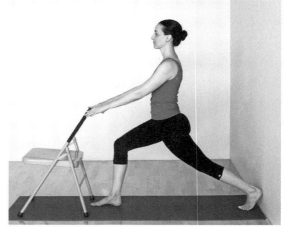

Crescent Warrior Pose with heel at wall and hands on chair

POSE INSTRUCTIONS

1. Place a chair on one end of the mat with back of the chair toward you.

2. Begin in Mountain Pose (see page 220 for instructions) with your hands on the back of the chair.

3. Bend your right knee and step your left foot back. Press your toes into the earth, straighten your left leg and lift your heel.

4. If necessary, position your left foot farther out to the left to adjust the stance for your balance.

5. Square your hips to the front of your mat by drawing your right hip back and your left hip forward.

6. Lift up and out of your waist, lengthening your sides.

7. Draw your belly in and up as you lengthen your tailbone down.

8. Lift one OR both of your arms straight overhead in line with your ears, and draw your shoulder blades together on your back.

9. Lengthen the back of your neck, and gaze past your nose.

10. Enjoy Crescent Warrior Pose for 3 to 5 breaths.

11. Return to Mountain Pose.

12. Practice the instructions above using the opposite side of your body.

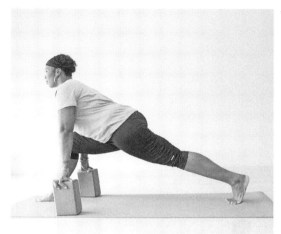
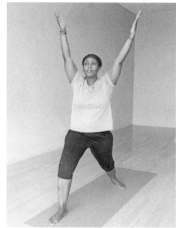

Crescent Warrior Pose as lunge with blocks   Warrior 1 Pose

ADAPTATIONS AND VARIATIONS

- Practice Crescent Warrior Pose with heel against wall and hands on chair back in front of you.

- Practice Crescent Warrior Pose without the support of a chair.

- Practice Crescent Warrior as a lunge:

  1. Begin in Table Pose (see page 280 for instructions), and have two blocks handy.

  2. Step your right foot forward and place blocks on either side of your right foot.

  3. Place hands on blocks and lift your left knee. Straighten your left leg as you press out through your heel.

  4. Draw your belly in, off your right thigh, and hug your legs together.

- Practice Crescent Pose in a Chair variations (see page 160 for instructions).

- Practice Crescent Kneeling Lunge Pose (see page 162 for instructions).

- Practice Warrior 1 Pose. It is different from Crescent Warrior Pose because the back heel is pivoted down on the earth. You may practice Warrior 1 Pose with hands on a chair against a wall, OR practice pose in the middle of your mat.

Dolphin Dog Pose (Downward Facing Dog on Forearms)

Adho Mukha Svanasana Variation

PRIMARY BENEFITS

▩ Strengthens upper body

▩ Lengthens spine

▩ Stretches shoulders, backs of legs, and arches of feet

PRECAUTIONS

▩ Shoulder or neck condition, injury, or pain

PROPS

▩ Yoga mat

▩ Chair

▩ Yoga block

▩ Wall

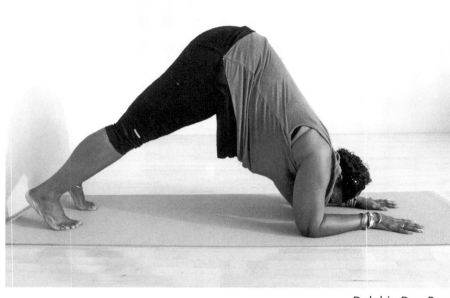

Dolphin Dog Pose

POSE INSTRUCTIONS

1. Begin in Table Pose (see page 280 for instructions).

2. Place your forearms parallel to one another on the mat with your elbows under your shoulders.

3. Press your forearms down and hug your elbows toward each other, energetically, without moving them.

4. Draw your shoulder blades together on your back.

5. Curl your toes under.

6. Draw your belly in and lift your knees off the mat.

7. Raise your hips skyward and straighten your legs to form an upside down "V" with your body. Your heels may or may not touch the earth.

8. Lengthen your tailbone down toward your heels.

9. Draw your shoulder blades together down your back.

10. Lengthen the back of your neck by gazing at your hands.

11. Enjoy Dolphin Dog Pose for 3 to 5 breaths.

12. Lower into Table Pose.

ADAPTATIONS AND VARIATIONS

- Practice with knees bent.
- Interlace your fingers instead of placing your forearms parallel to one another.
- Hug a yoga block between your forearms OR hands.
- Practice Dolphin Dog Pose with a chair against a wall. Interlace your fingers and place forearms on chair.
- Practice Sphinx Pose at the wall (see page 266 for instructions).
- Practice Table Pose on forearms (see page 280 for instructions).

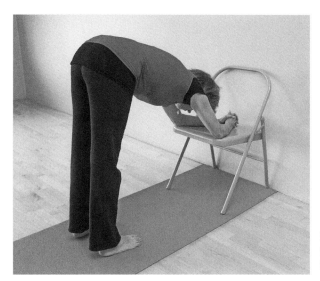

Dolphin Dog Pose on forearms with chair, fingers interlaced

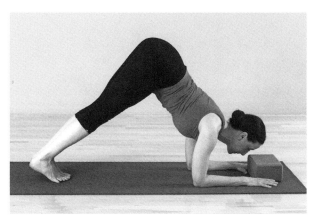

Dolphin Dog Pose with block corners held between index fingers and thumbs

Downward Facing Dog Pose

Adho Mukha Svanasana

PRIMARY BENEFITS

▣ Strengthens and lengthens spine, legs, and arms

▣ Opens shoulders

▣ Energizes mind and body

PRECAUTIONS

▣ Spine, shoulder, wrist, knee condition, injury, or pain

▣ Pregnancy

▣ Carpel Tunnel Syndrome

PROPS

▣ Yoga mat

▣ Yoga block

▣ Yoga dumbbells

▣ Rolled mat or wedge

▣ Wall

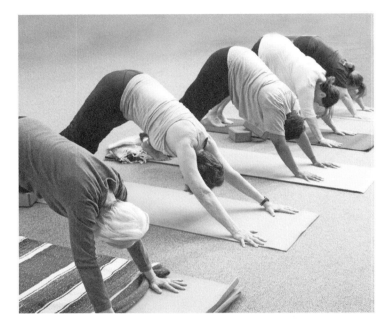

Downward Facing Dog Pose

POSE INSTRUCTIONS

1. Begin in Table Pose (see page 280 for instructions).
2. Draw your shoulder blades together onto your back, and press your hands into the earth. Make sure you root your index finger knuckles and your thumbs.
3. Curl your toes under.
4. Draw your belly in and lift your knees off the mat.
5. Raise your hips skyward and straighten your legs to form an upside "V" with your body. Your heels may or may not touch the earth.
6. Lengthen your tailbone down toward your heels.
7. Draw your shoulder blades together down your back.
8. Lengthen the back of your neck by gazing at your hands.
9. Enjoy Downward Facing Dog Pose for 3 to 5 breaths. Lower into Table Pose.

ADAPTATIONS AND VARIATIONS

• Practice with knees bent.

- Place a wedge or rolled mat under your wrists, OR use yoga dumbbells.
- Practice with a block between your thighs.
- Place a block on the earth and rest your forehead on it.
- If your hamstrings and lower back muscles are tight, bend your knees and angle your hips high to find the lower back curve. Then slowly straighten your legs while maintaining the lower back curve.
- Practice Downward Facing Dog Pose with one leg lifted.
- Practice Wall Dog or Wall Dog with a chair (see page 305 for instructions).

I have learned how to get down to the floor, and how to get up again too, using Downward Dog. I even practiced this pose after slipping on an ice patch!

CONNIE, YOGA MOVES STUDENT

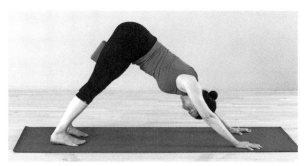

Downward Facing Dog Pose with block between thighs

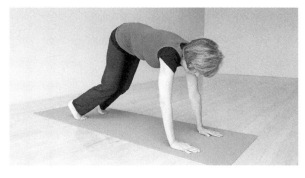

Downward Facing Dog Pose with knees bent

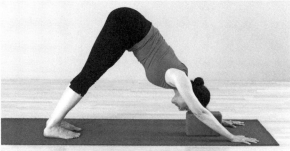

Downward Facing Dog Pose with block under forehead

Eagle Pose in a Chair

Garudasana Variation

PRIMARY BENEFITS

■ Opens area between shoulder blades

■ Opens outer hips and thighs

■ Strengthens legs, knees, and ankles

PRECAUTIONS

■ Spine, shoulder, wrist, hip, knee, or ankle condition, injury, or pain

PROPS

■ Yoga mat

■ Chair

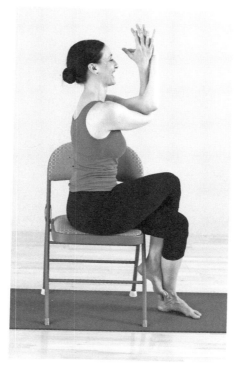 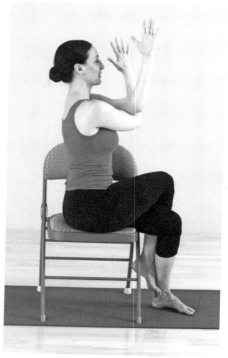

Eagle Pose in a Chair   Eagle Pose in a Chair, forearms apart

POSE INSTRUCTIONS

1. Position yourself sitting sideways in a chair, with the left side of your body facing the back of the chair.

2. Cross your right thigh over your left thigh to stack your knees and hug your legs together. Your ankles may or may not intertwine by hooking the top of your right foot behind your left calf or ankle.

3. Straighten your arms in front of you at shoulder height. Bend your elbows so that your fingers are pointing skyward and hands face each other.

4. Cross your right elbow underneath your left elbow.

5. The back of your hands and forearms should now be facing each other. This is Eagle Pose with forearms apart.

6. For the full pose, continue wrapping your forearms and wrists until you can claps hands, OR your right fingers can press into the mound of your left thumb.

7. Lift your elbows as high as you can.

8. Tuck your chin slightly as your upper back rounds and you breathe into the back of your ribs and shoulder blades. Pull your belly in and up.

9. Enjoy Eagle Pose in a Chair for 3 to 5 breaths.

10. Practice the instructions above using the opposite leg and arm.

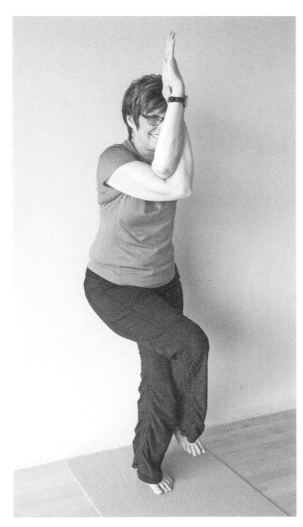

Eagle Pose
against wall

Eagle Pose in a Chair

ADAPTATIONS AND VARIATIONS

- Practice Eagle Pose standing against a wall OR standing in the center of a mat, for balance practice. You may touch your right toes to the earth when the right leg is wrapped around the left leg.

- Practice the arm portion of pose OR the leg portion of pose separately.

- Practice Eagle Pose arms variation. Cross arms at your wrists, with palms facing away from each other, and at throat level.

- Practice Half-Eagle Pose seated on the earth. Begin in Stick Pose (see page 276 for instructions). Keep your left leg straight, then bend and cross the right knee over the left knee, stacking the knees over or toward each other. Press the top of your right foot onto the earth. Place "spider" hands on either side of your hips and gently lean forward.

- Practice Yoga Moves Your Core, Variation 4: Eagle Pose Curls (see page 92 for instructions).

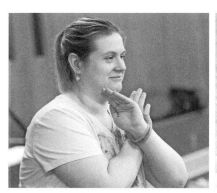
Eagle Pose arm variation

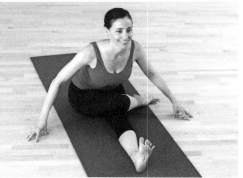
Half-Eagle Pose on earth

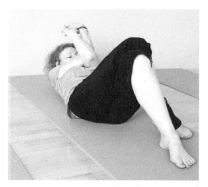
Eagle Pose Curl

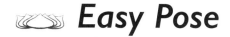 # *Easy Pose*

Sukhasana

PRIMARY BENEFITS

■ Provides comfortable seated position for rest, centering, breath, and meditation practice

■ Strengthens core and back

PRECAUTIONS

■ Knee, hip, or spinal condition, injury, or pain

PROPS

■ Yoga mat

■ Yoga block

■ Blankets

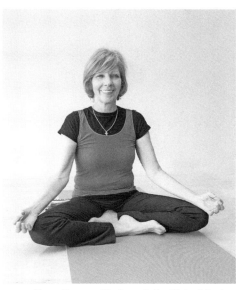 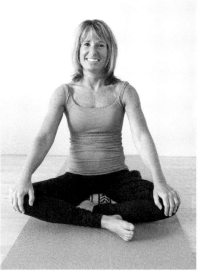

Easy Pose with hands in Chin Mudra   Easy Pose on blanket

POSE INSTRUCTIONS

1. Begin in Stick Pose (see page 276 for instructions).

2. Bend your left knee and place your left heel next to your groin.

3. Bend your right knee and place your right heel on the outside of your left foot or ankle.

4. Press your hands into the earth to lift your hips. Tilt the top of your pelvis forward and rest your hips back to the earth, keeping a slight curve in the low back.

5. Sit tall with your spine erect, and your neck and head in line with your spine, as though a puppet string is being pulled from the top of your head.

6. Rest your outstretched hands on your knees with palms facing down, OR facing up, OR with hands in Chin Mudra (see page 328 for instructions).

7. Soften your skin, jaw, and tongue.

8. Enjoy and rest comfortably in Easy Pose for 3 to 5 breaths or more, depending on whether your intention is to practice the yoga posture or to use the posture for *pranayama* (breathing) or meditation practice.

Easy Pose

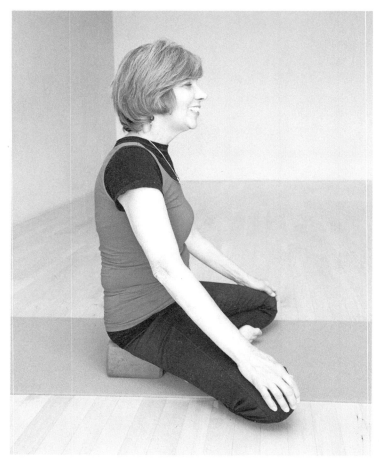

Easy Pose sitting on block

ADAPTATIONS AND VARIATIONS

- Place a yoga block or blankets under your buttocks for a neutral pelvis, and to ensure your knees are at hip height or lower.
- Place a block under each knee for comfort in the pose.
- Fold your legs into a comfortable cross-legged position.
- Place one hand on your belly and one hand on your heart as you breath.
- Practice various Breathing Practices (see page 28 for instructions) while in Easy Pose.
- Meditate in Easy Pose.

Extended Side Angle Pose in a Chair

Utthita Parsvakonasana Variation

PRIMARY BENEFITS

■ Lengthens sides of body

■ Opens hips

■ Strengthens your core, hips, and legs

■ Improves balance

PRECAUTIONS

■ Shoulder, hip, or knee condition, injury, or pain

PROPS

■ Yoga mat

■ Yoga block

■ 1 to 2 chairs

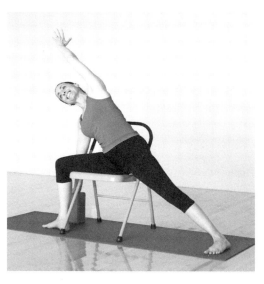

Extended Side Angle Pose in a Chair with right hand on block

POSE INSTRUCTIONS

1. Place a chair in the center of your mat facing the long side, with a block handy.

2. Begin in Mountain Pose in a Chair (see page 222 for instructions), sitting slightly forward on the edge of the seat.

3. Widen your right leg to the right with your toes and knee pointing toward the short edge of the mat. Place your heel under your knee with the center of your kneecap aligned with the middle toe.

4. Straighten the left leg out to the left side with your foot pressing into the earth and your toes facing the long side of the mat.

5. Place your right forearm on your right thigh and draw your shoulder blades together on your back.

6. Straighten your left arm over your ear and reach to the right. Gaze forward OR at your fingertips.

7. Feel the stretch along the left side of your body from your hips to your fingers.

8. Enjoy Extended Side Angle Pose in a Chair for 3 to 5 breaths.

9. Practice the instructions above using the opposite side of your body.

Extended Side Angle Pose in a Chair

ADAPTATIONS AND VARIATIONS

- Place your right hand on a block, OR on the earth outside your right ankle.

- Practice Extended Side Angle Pose with two chairs. Place your right forearm on a second chair placed on your right side. Make sure your right shoulder is over your elbow.

- Practice by only moving your bent right leg to the right side, while keeping your left knee bent and in front of you. Your legs will form a right angle.

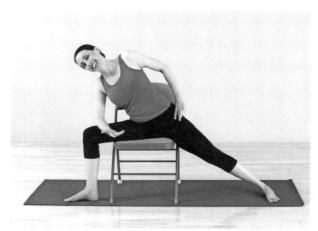

Extended Side Angle
Pose in a Chair with
forearm on thigh
and left hand on hip

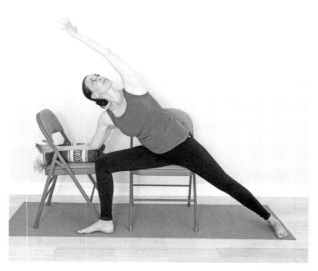

Extended Side Angle
Pose with two chairs
and forearm on blanket
on second chair

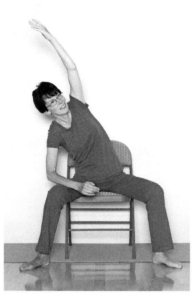

Extended Side Angle Pose in a Chair with both knees bent as in Goddess Pose

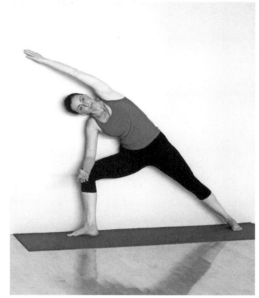

Extended Side Angle Pose against wall

- Practice the pose with legs as in Goddess Pose (see page 187 for photo). Place a chair between your thighs to help keep legs apart.

- To keep both shoulder blades engaged on the back, you can first straighten your left arm along the left side of your body pointing toward your left toes. Second, bend your left elbow with the thumb pointing toward your shoulder and hug your upper arm into you body. Third, straighten your left arm over your ear and reach to the right.

- Practice Extended Side Angle Pose with one buttock on the chair. Grasp the chair seat with both hands. Keeping your right sitting bone and thigh on the chair while moving your left sitting bone off the left side of the chair. Extend the left leg to the side.

- Practice Extended Side Angle Pose in the middle of your mat.

Fire Log Pose

Agnistambhasana

PRIMARY BENEFITS

■ Opens hips and inner groin muscles

PRECAUTIONS

■ Knee, hip, or spine condition, injury, or pain

PROPS

■ Yoga mat

■ Blanket

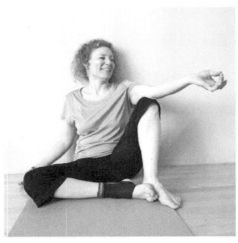

Todd's "By the Beach" Pose

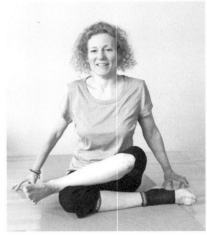

Fire Log Pose

POSE INSTRUCTIONS

1. Begin seated on the earth with your knees bent skyward and your feet flat.

2. Place your right knee down to the earth with your right foot next to your left ankle.

3. Lean into your right hip and hand. This can be enough of a stretch. If so, place your left elbow on your left knee and your fingers in Chin Mudra (see page 328 for instructions). Pretend you are on the beach enjoying the view. We call this Todd's "By the Beach" Pose. This might be enough, or you can continue with the instructions.

4. You may choose to stack your shins to achieve the full Fire Log Pose. Roll toward your right, lifting your left hip, and stack your left shin over your right shin so that the left foot is over and beyond the right knee. Lower your left hip so your weight is balanced on both hips.

5. Enjoy holding Fire Log Pose for 3 to 5 breaths.

6. Practice the instructions above using the opposite side of the body.

ADAPTATIONS AND VARIATIONS

- Practice Fire Log Pose preparation against the wall with "cactus" arms.

- Place a blanket under your knee or ankle for comfort and support.

- Practice Half Fire Log Pose. Begin in Stick Pose (see page 276 for instructions). Cross your right ankle over your left thigh. Tilt your pelvis forward for a gentle stretch. Enjoy for 3 to 5 breaths. You may place a blanket under your hips for a neutral pelvis.

- Begin seated with knees bent and place your hands behind your hips. Place left foot close to left buttock. Cross right ankle over your left knee and flex your right foot. Move your buttocks closer to your left foot until you feel the stretch in your right hip. Enjoy for 3 to 5 breaths.

- Practice #4 Pose (see page 130 for instructions) on the earth or in a chair.

- Practice Pigeon Pose (see page 227 for instructions).

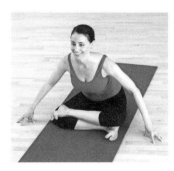

Fire Log Pose

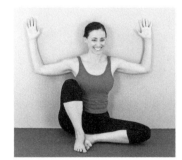

Preparation for Fire Log Pose against wall with "cactus" arms

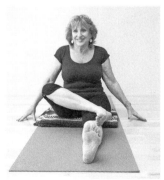

Half Fire Log Pose

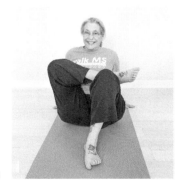

Fire Log Pose Variation

Forward Fold Pose

Uttanasana

PRIMARY BENEFITS

■ Stretches spine, hamstrings, and calves

■ Releases tension

■ Quiets the mind and draws you inward

PRECAUTIONS

■ Spine, neck, hip, hamstring, or knee condition, injury, or pain

■ Sciatica

■ Balance concerns

PROPS

■ Yoga mat

■ Yoga block

■ Wall

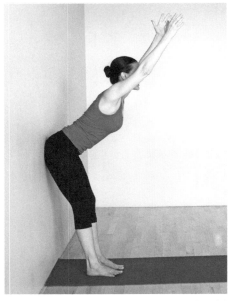

Partial Forward Fold
Pose with soft knees

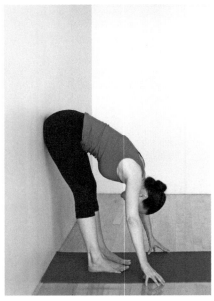

Forward Fold Pose

POSE INSTRUCTIONS

1. Begin in Mountain Pose (see page 220 for instructions) with your hips against a wall and your feet about a foot away from the wall.

2. Lift your arms skyward and feel your shoulder blades draw together on your back.

3. Leading with your heart, hinge from your hips, and begin to lean your spine forward while keeping your hips against the wall, and your knees softened.

4. Slowly lower your hands to the earth.

5. Press your fingertips firmly into the earth.

6. Lengthen your tailbone down toward your heels, and draw your belly in and up.

7. Look between your legs and release neck tension.

8. Enjoy Forward Fold for 3 to 5 breaths.

9. Place your hands on your hips, press down through your feet, lead with your heart, and rise slowly with a straight spine and your shoulder blades drawn together on your back.

ADAPTATIONS AND VARIATIONS

- If you cannot reach the earth, bend your knees slightly until you can, as long as your spine remains straight.
- Practice with your hands on your hips, OR out to the side in a "T" position.
- Place fingertips on blocks or a chair to raise the earth to your hands.
- Practice with fingers interlaced behind your back, OR holding opposite elbows in front.
- Practice Forward Fold Pose in the middle of the mat.
- Practice Forward Fold Pose in a Chair (see page 185 for instructions).
- Practice Restorative Forward Fold (see page 247 for instructions).
- Practice Stick Pose forward fold variation (see page 278 for instructions).
- Practice Wide Angle Forward Fold Pose, Variation 3 (see page 316 for instructions).

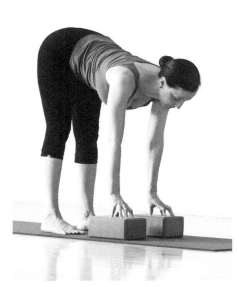

Forward Fold Pose with fingertips on block

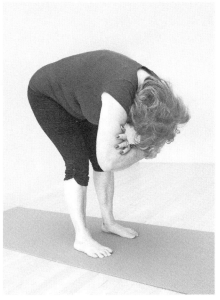

Forward Fold Pose with bent knees and holding opposite elbows

Forward Fold Pose

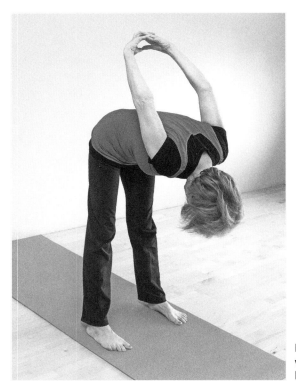

Forward Fold Pose
with fingers interlaced
behind back

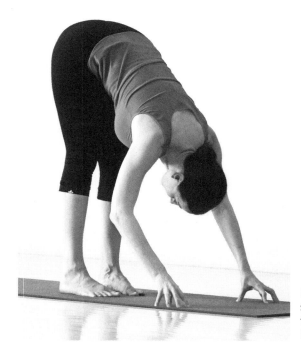

Forward Fold Pose
standing with
fingertips pressing
into mat

Forward Fold Pose in a Chair

Uttanasana Variation

PRIMARY BENEFITS

- Stretches spine
- Releases tension
- Quiets mind and draws you inward

PRECAUTIONS

- Spine, neck, hip condition, injury, or pain

PROPS

- Yoga mat
- Yoga block
- 1 or 2 chairs

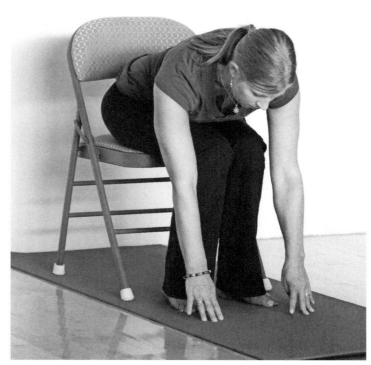

Forward Fold Pose in a Chair

POSE INSTRUCTIONS

1. Begin in Mountain Pose in a Chair (see page 222 for instructions).
2. Lift your arms skyward and hug your shoulder blades together on your back.
3. Leading with your heart, hinge from your hips and begin to lean your spine forward.
4. Slowly lower your arms to the earth OR a block.
5. Press your fingertips firmly into the earth.
6. Lengthen your tailbone down toward the earth, and draw your belly in and up.

Forward Fold Pose in a Chair

7. Look at your feet, OR between your legs to release neck tension.

8. Enjoy Forward Fold Pose in a Chair for 3 to 5 breaths.

9. Place your hands on your hips, press down through the back of your thighs and feet, and rise slowly with a straight spine.

ADAPTATIONS AND VARIATIONS

- Practice Forward Fold Pose in a Chair with your hands around your shins and holding opposite elbows, OR your arms out to the side in a "T" position.

- Practice Forward Fold Pose with two chairs with your legs and arms extended on a second chair in front of you.

- Practice Forward Fold Pose (see page 182 for instructions).

- Practice Restorative Forward Fold Pose (see page 247 for instructions).

- Practice Stick Pose (see page 276 for instructions).

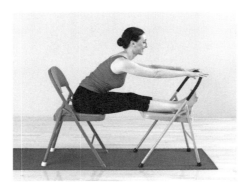

Forward Fold Pose with two chairs

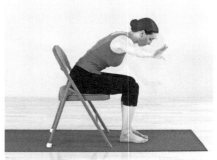

Forward Fold Pose in a Chair with arms in "T"

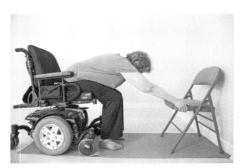

Forward Fold Pose with two chairs

Goddess Pose in a Chair

Deviasana

PRIMARY BENEFITS

■ Opens inner thighs and hips

■ Strengthens thighs

■ Strengthens calves and arches with addition of heel lifts

■ Opens shoulders with arm positions

PRECAUTIONS

■ Inner thigh, ankle, knee, or shoulder condition, injury, or pain

PROPS

■ Yoga mat

■ Chair

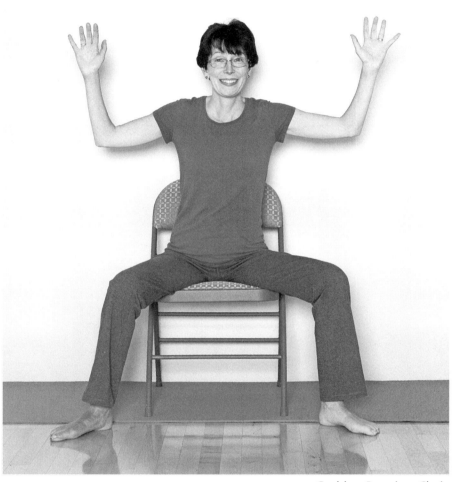

Goddess Pose in a Chair

POSE INSTRUCTIONS

1. Begin in Mountain Pose in a Chair (see page 222 for instructions).
2. Place your feet wide and open both knees out to the sides.
3. Track your knees over your middle toes with heels under your knees.
4. Place your arms in "cactus" position.
5. Enjoy Goddess Pose for 3 to 5 breaths.

Goddess Pose in a Chair

ADAPTATIONS AND VARIATIONS

- Practice Goddess Pose with hands on thighs.
- If inner thighs are tight, open one knee to the side, with the other pointing straight ahead.
- Practice Goddess Pose with arms in Eagle Pose position (see page 172 for instructions).
- Practice Goddess Pose with a side bend. After step 3 above, place your right forearm on your right thigh, raise your left arm over your head and reach to your right. Press your left hip into the chair as you reach and feel the stretch along your left side.
- Lift your heels and arches, and spread your toes.
- Practice Goddess Pose with two chairs facing each other. Follow pose instructions above and place a second chair between your thighs to keep them wide. You may make them wider still by inserting blocks between chair and thighs.

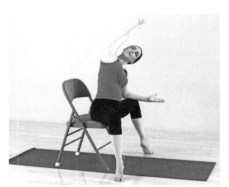

Goddess Pose in a Chair with side bend and heels lifted

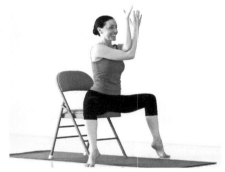

Goddess Pose in a Chair with Eagle Pose arms and heels lifted

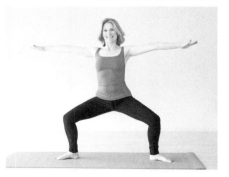

Goddess Pose in middle of mat

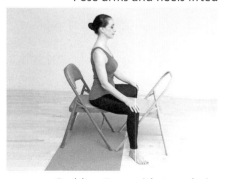

Goddess Pose with two chairs

Half Lord of the Fishes Pose

Ardha Matsyendrasana

PRIMARY BENEFITS

▓ Increases spinal flexibility

▓ Opens shoulders and hips

▓ Improves sciatica

▓ Improves digestion

PRECAUTIONS

▓ Neck, shoulder, spinal, or knee condition, injury, or pain

PROPS

▓ Yoga mat

▓ Yoga block

▓ Blanket

▓ 1 to 2 chairs

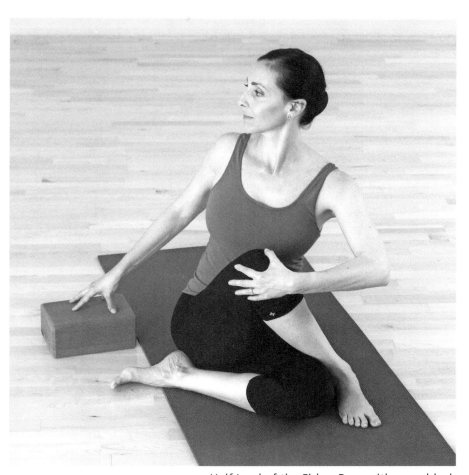

Half Lord of the Fishes Pose with yoga block

POSE INSTRUCTIONS

1. Begin seated on the earth with your knees bent skyward and your feet flat.

2. Place your left foot under your right thigh and close to the right hip.

3. Leave your right foot as is, OR step it outside your left knee. Feel the sensation of the sole of your right foot pressing into the earth. Your right knee should be pointing skyward.

4. Interlace your fingers around your right shin and lift your heart skyward as you inhale.

Half Lord of the Fishes Pose

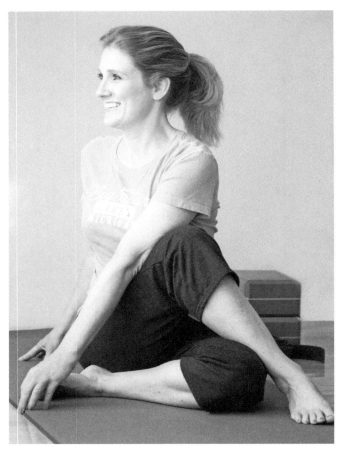

Half Lord of the
Fishes Pose with
elbow outside thigh

5. Keeping your left hand around your right knee and your spine long, place your right fingertips behind your right hip and press into the earth as you exhale.

6. Begin the twist from your navel and then continue the twist up your spine.

7. Roll your right shoulder back.

8. Turn your head toward the right after you have twisted your spine. Turning your head too far to the right may strain your neck.

9. Enjoy Half Lord of the Fishes Pose for 3 to 5 breaths.

10. Practice instructions above using the opposite side of your body.

ADAPTATIONS AND VARIATIONS

- Place a folded blanket under both hips.
- Place your right fingertips on the block.
- If your right hip is not touching the earth, place a folded blanket under the left hip.
- To enjoy a shoulder opener in the pose, place your left elbow on the outside of your right thigh, press the thigh and elbow into each other.
- Practice Half Lord of the Fishes Pose with the left leg extended.
- Practice Half Lord of the Fishes Pose on one or two chairs.
- Practice a twist seated in Easy Pose (see page 175 for instructions).
- Practice Sage Twist (see page 255 for instructions).
- Practice Spinal Twist in a Chair (see page 271 for instructions).

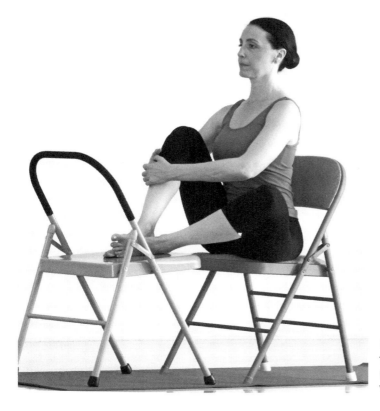

Half Lord of
the Fishes Pose
preparation
with two chairs

Half Moon Pose

Ardha Chandrasana

PRIMARY BENEFITS

▓ Improves balance

▓ Strengthens spine, hips, legs, and abdominals

▓ Opens shoulders, hamstrings, and inner groin muscles

PRECAUTIONS

▓ Balance concerns

▓ Neck, spine, shoulder, hip, or knee condition, injury, or pain

PROPS

▓ Yoga mat

▓ Yoga block

▓ Chair

▓ Blanket

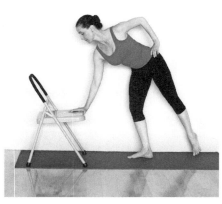

Half Moon Pose preparation with front knee bent

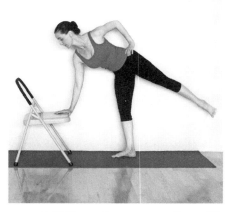

Half Moon Pose preparation with back leg partially lifted

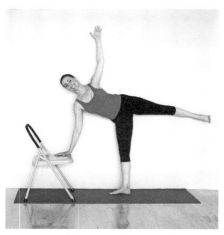

Half Moon Pose against wall with lower hand on chair

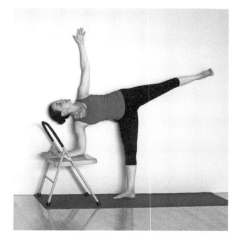

Half Moon Pose against wall with forearm on chair

POSE INSTRUCTIONS

1. Place a mat lengthwise against a wall and place a chair at the right end (when your back is to the wall).

2. Stand in center of the mat with your back against the wall.

3. Place your right hand OR forearm on the chair.

4. Place your left hand on your hip.

5. Push off the earth with your left foot, lifting it to hip height.

6. Roll your left shoulder blade onto your back and toward the wall.

7. Stack your shoulders vertically, one over the other, and stack your hips one over the other.

8. Flex your left foot.

9. Press down to the earth with your right foot, especially through the mound of your right big toe. Tone your right buttocks. At the same time, draw energy up from the earth through your standing leg. Be careful not to lock your knee.

10. Rise up and out of the lower hip as you extend your tailbone down toward your heel.

11. Lift your left arm skyward and gaze forward OR toward your left finger tips.

12. Enjoy Half Moon Pose for 3 to 5 breaths.

13. Practice instructions above using the opposite side of your body.

ADAPTATIONS AND VARIATIONS

- Place blankets under your forearm on the chair.
- Reach your right fingertips to a yoga block, OR on the earth.
- Practice Half Moon Pose in the middle of the mat.
- Practice Spinal Balance Pose (see page 268 for instructions).

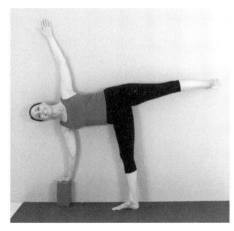

Half Moon Pose against wall with block beneath lower arm

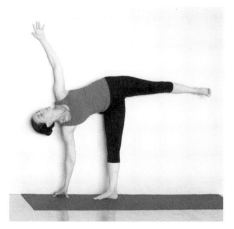

Half Moon Pose against wall

Handstand Pose on the Earth

Adho Mukha Vrksasana Variation

PRIMARY BENEFITS

■ Strengthens upper body

■ Improves mood and confidence

■ Uses creativity and imagination

■ Improves balance

PRECAUTIONS

■ Shoulder, elbow or wrist condition, injury, or pain

PROPS

■ Yoga mat

■ Yoga strap

■ Wall

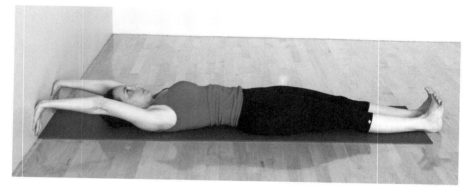

Handstand Pose on the Earth

POSE INSTRUCTIONS

1. Place the short end of your mat at the wall.

2. Begin in Mountain Pose on the Earth (see page 221 for instructions) with your head toward the wall, and arm length from the wall.

3. Lengthen your arms overhead, and press your palms into the wall.

4. Flex your feet, and press your thighs down into the mat.

5. Draw your lower ribs down toward the earth. Pull your belly in and up, and lengthen your tailbone down toward your heels.

6. Visualize standing on your hands, with your feet extending skyward, reversing your daily upright stance.

7. Enjoy Handstand Pose on the Earth for 5 to 10 breaths.

ADAPTATIONS AND VARIATIONS

• Have a friend assist you with Handstand Pose on the Earth. A friend may help you feel sensations of the pose by touching the ankles, OR pressing into your feet OR heels, as you continue to press your hands overhead into the wall. You may also press your feet into your friend's hands for greater sensation.

• Practice Handstand Pose standing on your feet. Begin in Mountain Pose (see page 220 for instructions) and lift your arms straight overhead with palms pressing skyward. Imagine being in this pose with your body inverted: your hands would press into the earth while your feet would press toward the sky.

- Practice Downward Facing Dog Pose with one leg lifted skyward. Begin in Downward Facing Dog (see page 170 for instructions). Lift your right leg skyward for 3 breaths.

- Practice Wall Dog Pose (see page 305 for instructions).

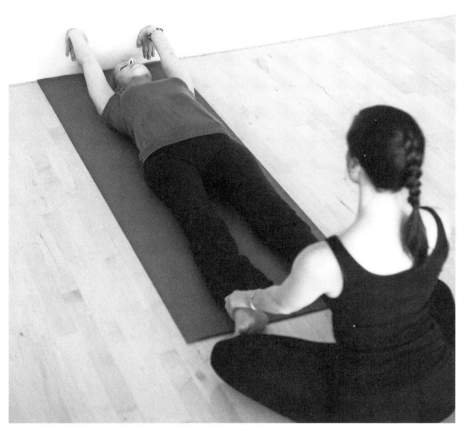

Handstand Pose on the Earth with partner
gently pressing on ankles

Happy Baby Pose

Ananda Balasana

PRIMARY BENEFITS

■ Stretches groin muscles, inner thighs, and back

■ Opens hips

■ Massages back of spine

■ Lifts mood with a sense of play

PRECAUTIONS

■ Neck, shoulder, or knee condition, injury, or pain

PROPS

■ Yoga mat

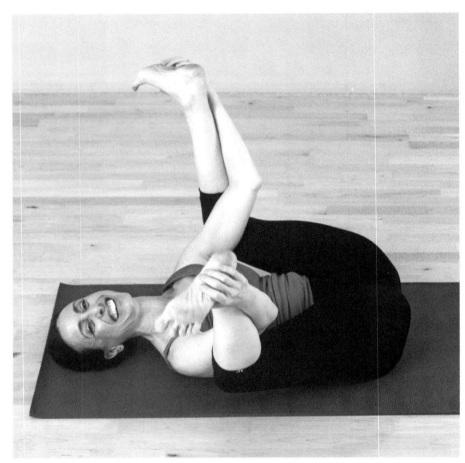

Happy Baby Pose with hands on outside of feet

POSE INSTRUCTIONS

1. Begin in Bridge Prep Pose (see page 137 for instructions).

2. Raise your knees into your heart and grasp your feet, ankles, OR calves. You may reach for them either on the outside or inside of your legs.

3. Flex and separate your feet, raise them skyward, and draw your thighs toward your shoulders.

4. Roll gently to one side and then the other, back and forth.

5. Enjoy rolling in the Happy Baby Pose for 3 to 5 breaths.

ADAPTATIONS AND VARIATIONS

- Place a blanket under your head.

- To intensify the stretch and to build strength, press your hands into the bottom of your feet and your feet into your hands.

- Practice Happy Baby Pose with leg resistance, known as "Dead Bug" Pose. Release your hands, and flex your wrist with palms skyward. Press your upper arms into your thighs and your lower arms into your calves while your legs press against your arms. Exhale as you pull your belly in toward your spine and your chin to your chest. Hold for 3 to 5 breaths.

Yoga is a gift you give yourself. Practicing yoga is the one time YOU have control of your body and mind. I have learned through yoga that I can be in control. The mind-body connection is indisputable. Yoga takes me to my happy place.

BETSY, YOGA MOVES STUDENT

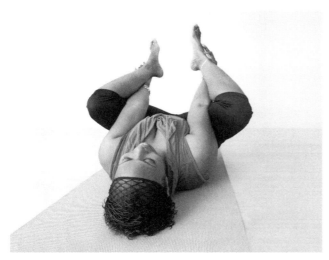

Happy Baby Pose with arms woven inside legs and wrapped around ankles and feet

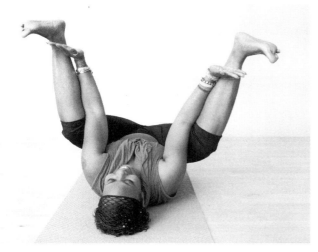

"Dead Bug" Pose

Headstand Pose Variations

Salamba Sirsasana

PRIMARY BENEFITS

■ Calms, centers, and uplifts mood

■ Strengthens shoulder girdle, upper body, and abdominal core

■ Stimulates heart and circulation, and provides fresh oxygen rich blood to brain

PRECAUTIONS

■ Spine, shoulder, neck, elbow, or wrist condition, injury, or pain

■ Balance concerns

PROPS

■ Yoga mat

■ Yoga block

■ Chair

■ Wall

The traditional headstand is considered by many as "the preserver of youth," and a remedy for a wide variety of conditions. The traditional headstand is a complex, advanced pose and should not be attempted without consulting your physician and with the assistance of a qualified yoga instructor. The variations below offer many benefits without the risks of standing on your head.

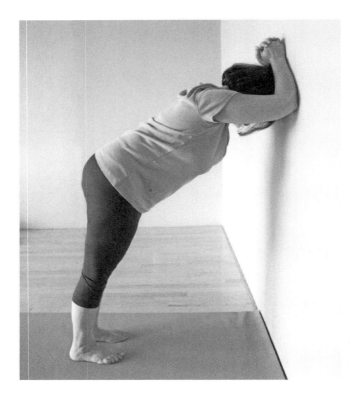

Variation 1:
Standing Headstand
Pose at raised angle

POSE INSTRUCTIONS

VARIATION 1: STANDING HEADSTAND POSE

1. Begin in Mountain Pose (see page 220 for instructions) facing the wall.

2. Interlace your fingers with their webbing snug but with loose rather than clenched fingers.

3. Place your elbows on the wall at shoulder height and shoulder distance apart.

4. Press your forearms and outsides of your wrists into the wall, making an inverted "V" with your arms.

5. Walk your feet back so there is a bend at the waist. As your forearms press into the wall, your hips will press away from the wall and the body will begin to look like an "L".

6. Draw your shoulder blades together onto your back, pull your belly in and up and lengthen your tailbone down.

7. Lengthen the top of your head toward the wall with a long neck. If the top of your head or hairline can touch the wall, gently press the crown into the wall in a way that allows you to maintain both the natural curve of your neck and your shoulder blades on your back.

8. Enjoy Standing Headstand Pose for 3 to 5 breaths or more. The longer you comfortably stay in the pose, the stronger you will become.

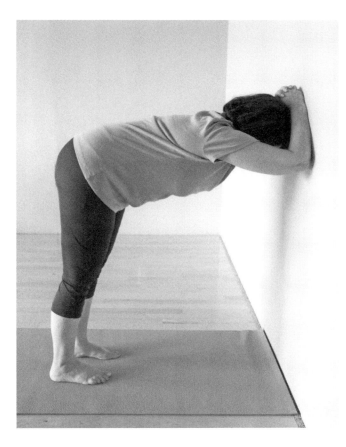

Variation 1:
Standing Headstand
Pose at right angle

Headstand Pose Variations

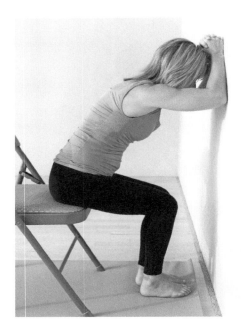

Variation 2:
Headstand Pose
in a Chair against
the wall

VARIATION 2: HEADSTAND POSE IN A CHAIR

1. Place a chair about 2 feet away from and facing the wall.

2. Begin in Mountain Pose in a Chair (see page 222 for instructions).

3. Interlace your fingers with their webbing snug but with loose rather than clenched fingers.

4. Leaning forward, place your elbows at shoulder height, and press your forearms and outsides of your wrists into the wall, making an inverted "V" with your arms.

5. Bring your shoulder blades onto your back, pull your belly in and up and lengthen your tailbone down.

6. Lengthen your spine through the back of your neck to the top of your head.

7. If the top of your head can touch the wall, gently press your crown into the wall in a way that allows you to maintain both the natural curve of your neck and your shoulder blades on your back.

8. Enjoy Headstand Pose in a Chair for 3 to 5 breaths or more. The longer you comfortably stay in the pose, the stronger you will become.

VARIATION 3: HEADSTAND POSE ON THE EARTH

1. Place the short edge of the mat to the wall.

2. Place a yoga block horizontally on the earth against the wall.

3. Begin in Bridge Prep Pose (see page 137 for instructions) with your head near the wall.

4. Place the top of your head against the block.

5. Bend your elbows and place your hands above your head and on the wall, with your fingers pointing toward the earth.

6. Use your legs for leverage, press your hands into the wall and the crown of your head gently against the block.

7. Slowly straighten your legs while continuing to press against the wall and block.

8. Visualize standing on your head. Energetically press out through your heels.

9. Enjoy Headstand Pose on the earth for 3 to 5 breaths or more.

VARIATION 4: DOLPHIN DOG POSE

(see page 168 for instructions).

VARIATION 5: FOREARM TABLE POSE

(see page 281 for instructions).

Yoga helps me to feel good about myself both physically and emotionally. It helps me to better accept the limitations from my MS. My balance, walking, coordination, and thinking are so much more positive after yoga

DAWN, YOGA MOVES STUDENT

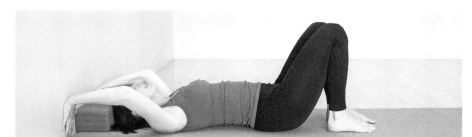

Variation 3: Headstand Pose on the Earth with bent knees

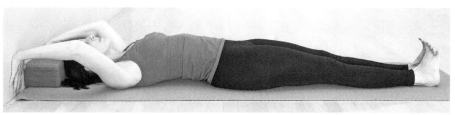

Variation 3: Headstand Pose on the Earth with straight legs

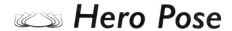 # *Hero Pose*

Virasana

PRIMARY BENEFITS

■ Stretches thighs, ankles, and feet

■ Strengthens arches

■ Neutralizes spine

■ Improves gait

PRECAUTIONS

■ Spine, knee, ankle, or foot condition, injury, or pain

PROPS

■ Yoga mat

■ Yoga block

■ Washcloths or small towels

■ Blanket(s)

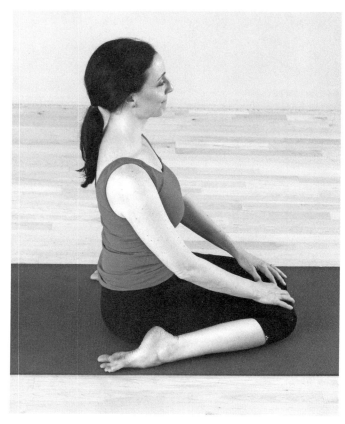

Hero Pose

POSE INSTRUCTIONS

1. Begin in Table Pose (see page 280 for instructions).

2. Bring you knees close together and angle your feet wider apart.

3. Lower your hips down between your inner heels and raise your torso upright.

4. Make sure your knees spread no wider than hip width apart.

5. If your sitting bones do not touch the earth, place a block OR a blanket under your sitting bones.

6. Press the tops of your feet into the earth and hug your heels toward your hips. Be careful not to let your heels roll out. Rest your hands on your knees.

7. Pull your belly in and up and lengthen your tailbone toward the earth.

8. Let gravity draw your inner thighs down as you lift your spine.

9. Enjoy Hero Pose for 3 to 5 breaths.

10. Return to Table Pose and stretch one leg straight back and then the other to lengthen the muscles behind your knees.

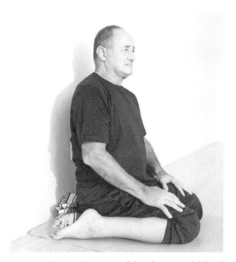

Hero Pose on blanket and block

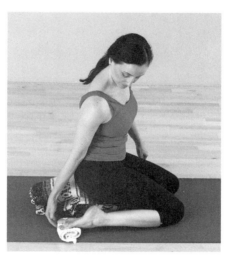

Hero Pose seated on blanket with washcloth under feet

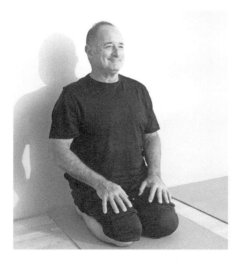

Thunderbolt Pose

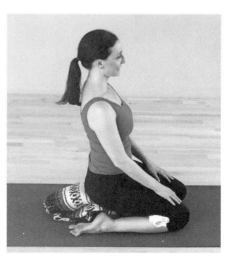

Hero Pose seated on blanket with washcloth behind knees

Hero Pose

ADAPTATIONS AND VARIATIONS

- Press fingers into heels and heels into fingers.

- To prevent foot cramps, place a washcloth or small towel between the top of your foot or ankle and the mat. You may wish to place a blanket under your knees as well.

- Before you sit back toward your heels, place your fingers behind your knees and lengthen your calf muscles toward your feet.

- To relieve knee discomfort, tuck a rolled washcloth between the back of your knee and your calf.

- For Half Hero Pose, extend the left leg in front of you and keep the right knee bent in the Hero Pose position. If needed, place a blanket or a block under the left hip to even your hips and/or under your left knee for comfort.

- Practice Thunderbolt Pose, a variation of Hero Pose, by sitting on your heels rather than between them. Your feet should be pointing straight back.

- For a deeper stretch and backbend from Hero Pose, begin to lean back onto your forearms and perhaps progress all the way down onto your back. Be sure to lengthen your tailbone toward your feet and draw your belly in and up to prevent lower back pain. Your knees should remain no wider than hip width apart.

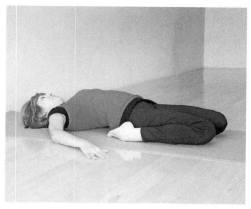

Hero Pose with backbend

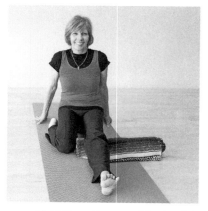

Half Hero Pose on block with blanket under knees

Inchworm Pose

PRIMARY BENEFITS

■ Loosens lower back and belly

■ Strengthens abdominal muscles

■ Conditions pelvic floor

■ Strengthens and tones lower back

PRECAUTIONS

■ Spinal injury

■ Pregnancy

PROPS

■ Yoga mat

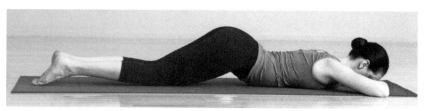

Inchworm Pose with pelvis tilted forward and tailbone lengthening toward heels

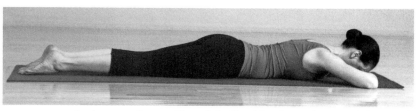

Inchworm Pose with pelvis tilted backward toward the earth

POSE INSTRUCTIONS

1. Begin on your belly. Stack your palms in front of you, and rest your forehead on the backs of your hands.

2. Tilt the top of your pelvis forward toward the earth as you tilt your sitting bones up toward the sky. There is space between your belly and the earth, and an arch in your lower spine.

3. Next, move the top of the pelvis backward toward the sky as you lengthen your sitting bones toward your heels. There is minimal space between the earth and your belly and your lower back is flattened.

4. Rock your pelvis forward on your inhale, and rock your pelvis backward on your exhale. Feel your belly fill on the inhale and softly contract on the exhale.

5. Repeat a round of rocking your pelvis as described above, matched with your inhales and exhales, 3 to 5 times.

ADAPTATIONS AND VARIATIONS

• Practice Cat and Cow Poses (see page 146 for instructions).

• Practice Cat and Cow Poses in a Chair (see page 148 for instructions).

• Practice Pelvic Tilts (see page 224 for instructions).

Leg Stretch Pose on the Back

Supta Padangusthasana

PRIMARY BENEFITS

■ Stretches hips, hamstrings, groin, inner thigh muscles, and calves

■ Reduces spasticity

■ Alleviates back pain

PRECAUTIONS

■ Knee, ankle, foot condition, injury, or pain

PROPS

■ Yoga mat

■ Yoga block

■ Yoga strap

■ Blanket

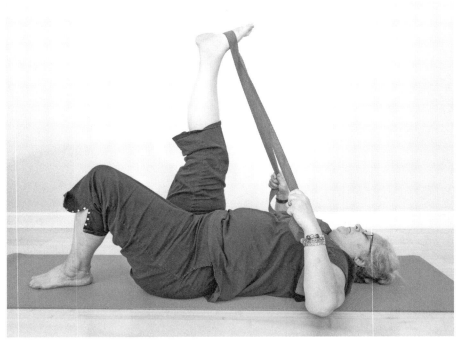

Leg Stretch Pose on the Back with yoga strap

POSE INSTRUCTIONS

1. Begin in Bridge Prep Prose (see page 137 for instructions).

2. Place a yoga strap around your right foot. Extend your right leg skyward. The knee should be directly over your hip even if your knee does not fully straighten.

3. Flex or "floint" your right foot so that your toes face toward you.

4. Pull your belly in and press your tailbone down.

5. Keep a firm, but not overly tight, grip on the yoga strap with one or both hands. Release any tension in your upper body, shoulders, neck and jaw.

6. Keeping your leg raised, press your thigh away from you until you feel a stretch in your calf or in your hamstrings.

7. Enjoy the Leg Stretch Pose for 3 to 5 breaths. You should feel the stretch in the middle of your hamstrings and calves. Refrain from stretching so strongly that you feel intense pain in your hamstring attachments or behind the knee.

8. Rotate your right leg in its hip socket so it angles toward your right shoulder. Extend it out to your right side and toward the floor until you feel a comfortable stretch in your inner thigh.

9. Pin your left hip down with your left hand to level your hips. Enjoy the stretch for 3 to 5 breaths.

10. Inhale, lift your leg back up to sky.

11. Exhale, and slowly release your leg down to the earth.

12. Notice the difference in how each leg feels, and then practice the instruction above using the opposite side of your body.

ADAPTATIONS AND VARIATIONS

• Place a blanket under your head to encourage a neutral neck curve.

• As you become more flexible, straighten the left leg for an even greater stretch. Press your left thigh into the earth, and extend a line of energy from your tailbone out through both heels.

• Place a yoga block between your foot and the strap and press your foot into the block.

Adaptive yoga is like no other form of exercise. It allows everyone to feel capable of doing anything. Can't do it that way, no problem, here's another way. It not only makes the body feel better, but there is a mental well-being that follows me after the practice of yoga. Whether you have limitations or not, we all need to adapt.

DEBORAH, YOGA MOVES STUDENT

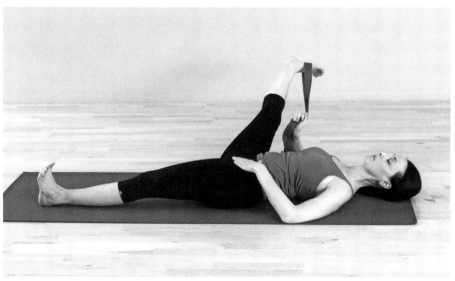

Leg Stretch Pose on the Back with external rotation and hand on hip

Leg Stretch Pose on the Back

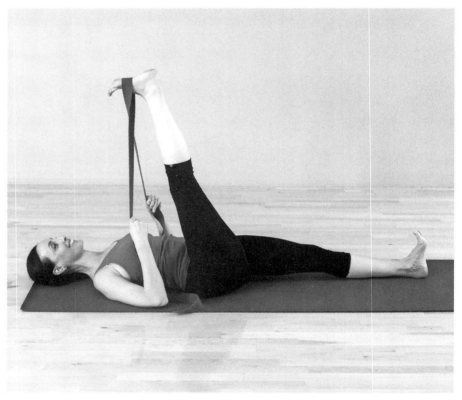

Leg Stretch Pose on the Back with left leg
extended and crossed strap on right foot

- Cross yoga strap in front of shin for easier grasping.
- When using a strap, experiment with its placement on your foot: it may be wrapped around the ball of the foot; OR the arch; OR the heel.
- Place a strap around your heel, cross it behind your calf and pull the strap toward you.
- In step 8, if your right leg is close to the floor, you can rest your right thigh on a block or blanket.
- Cross your right leg over your torso toward the left side of your body, and press through your heel. You may roll onto your left hip.
- Interlace your fingers behind your thigh instead of using a strap.

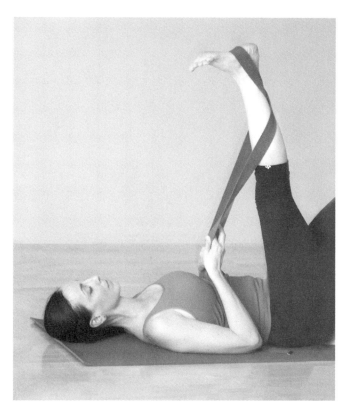

Leg Stretch Pose with yoga strap crossed behind calf and held with soft grip

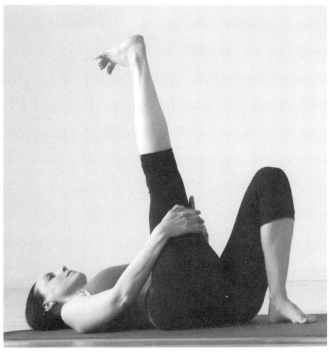

Leg Stretch Pose with interlaced fingers behind thigh and left knee bent

Leg Stretch Pose in a Chair

Padangusthasana Variation

PRIMARY BENEFITS

■ Stretches hips, hamstrings, groin, inner thighs and calves

■ Reduces spasticity

■ Relieves back pain

PRECAUTIONS

■ Hip, knee, foot condition, injury, or pain

PROPS

■ Yoga mat

■ Yoga strap

■ Chair

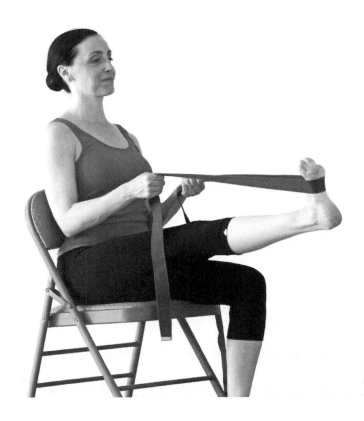

Leg Stretch Pose in a Chair with strap around the foot

POSE INSTRUCTIONS

1. Begin in Mountain Pose in a Chair (see page 222 for instructions).

2. Place a strap under the arch of your right foot.

3. Pull the strap in both hands to lift your knee hip height or higher.

4. Be careful not to hold the strap too tight; this will transfer unnecessary tension to your fingers, arms, or shoulders.

5. Extend your right leg forward.

6. Lengthen your spine and stretch your heel away from you.

7. Flex or "floint" your right foot.

8. Focus on feeling the stretch on the back of your thighs and calves. Be careful not to lock your knee.

9. Enjoy Leg Stretch Pose in a Chair for 3 to 5 breaths.

ADAPTATIONS AND VARIATIONS

- In place of yoga strap, interlace your fingers behind your thigh at its midpoint, stretching your heel away from you.

- Sit on the edge of the chair with hands grasping the sides of the seat. Outstretch your legs and press your heels into the earth while flexing your feet.

- When using a strap, experiment with its placement on your foot: it may be wrapped around the ball of the foot; OR the arch; OR the heel. Notice where you feel the stretch in each position.

- Practice Leg Stretch Pose with two chairs facing each other. Lift your right leg on the chair facing you. Place a strap around your foot and pull to feel the leg stretch.

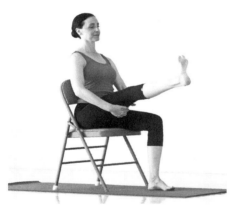

Leg Stretch Pose in a Chair with interlaced fingers behind thigh

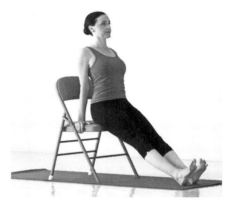

Leg Stretch Pose in a Chair with legs outstretched

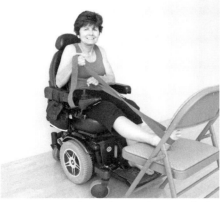

Leg Stretch Pose in two chairs and strap around foot

Legs Up the Wall Pose

Viparita Karani

PRIMARY BENEFITS

▧ Calms nervous system

▧ Reduces fatigue

▧ Increases energy

▧ Soothes heart

▧ Reduces fluid, swelling, and cramping in legs and feet

▧ Alleviates headaches

▧ Promotes restful sleep

▧ Reduces restless leg syndrome

▧ Reduces symptoms of menopause

PRECAUTIONS

▧ Do not practice this pose if you have:

  ▧ Glaucoma

  ▧ Neck pain or injury

  ▧ A hernia

  ▧ Hypertension

  ▧ A sinus infection

  ▧ Or are over 3 months pregnant

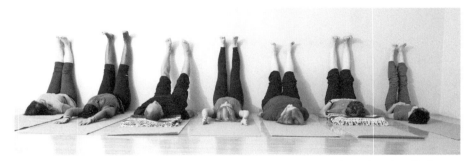

Legs Up the Wall Pose

Legs Up the Wall is the "Queen of Poses" for relieving stress and tension. It is said to be a preserver of youth. Many believe that this pose eases a variety of physical and emotional symptoms. This restorative pose also can be used in a more active way. Please note that getting into this pose takes some effort, but the enjoyment of Legs Up the Wall Pose is well worth it.

POSE INSTRUCTIONS

1. Place the short edge of your mat against the wall.

2. Begin seated next to the wall on the outside edge of the mat. Bend your knees. Place yourself sideways to the wall with right your hip as close to the wall as possible.

3. Slowly lean back to the earth. You may prop your elbow under your shoulder as you transition.

4. Swing your legs upward, and straighten them up the wall. You may use your hands to help raise your legs.

5. Make yourself comfortable by centering on the mat. Your arms can be on the earth, along your side, in "cactus" position, OR resting on your belly.

6. Enjoy Legs Up the Wall Pose as tolerated, and only 3 to 5 minutes when new to the pose, gradually working up to 20 minutes.

7. To come out of the pose, move slowly, lower your feet and roll to your right side into a fetal position. Remain on your side for several breaths before rising.

8. Once you have experience getting in and out of the pose, you will learn a way that works best for you.

Example 1

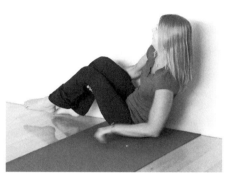

Preparation for Legs Up the Wall Pose Step 1

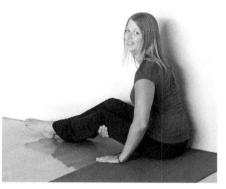

Preparation for Legs Up the Wall Pose Step 2

PROPS

- Yoga mat
- Yoga block
- Yoga strap
- Blanket(s)
- Bolster
- Wall
- Chair
- Eye mask
- Sandbags

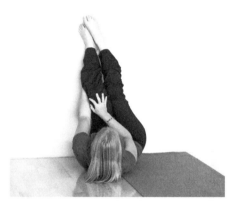

Preparation for Legs Up the Wall Pose Step 3

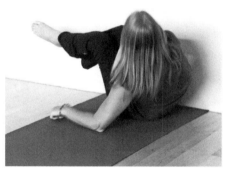

Preparation for Legs Up the Wall Pose Step 4

Example 2

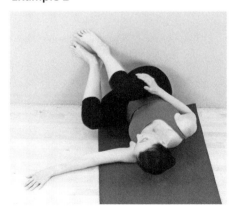

Preparation for Legs Up the Wall Pose Step 1

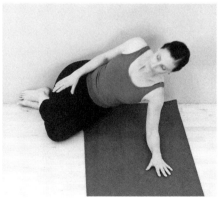

Preparation for Legs Up the Wall Pose Step 2

Legs Up the Wall Pose

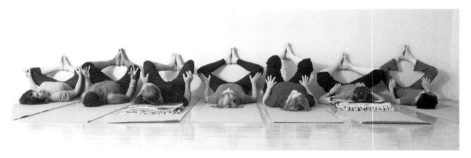

Legs Up the Wall Pose with "butterfly" legs

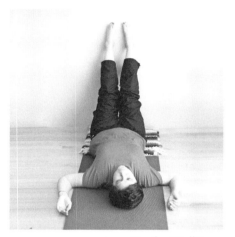

Legs Up the Wall Pose
with blanket under hips

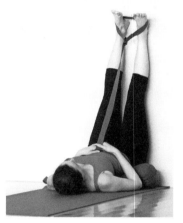

Legs Up the Wall Pose
with strap and bolster

ADAPTATIONS

- Place 1 to 2 blankets or a bolster under buttocks.
- If your head tilts back, place a blanket under it for a more neutral spine.
- If your legs need support to stay vertical, place a looped strap around your feet and hold the strap.
- Have a friend place a sandbag over the soles of your raised feet.
- Adjust how close your legs are to the wall, based on your flexibility and comfort. You may need to be further away from the wall and/or bend your knees, placing your feet on the wall.
- Practice Legs Up the Wall Pose with legs open into a "V" position.
- Practice Legs Up the Wall Pose with legs in "butterfly" position.

- If you feel tingling in your legs, bend your knees, and place your feet on the wall with your knees bent toward you, OR come out of the pose.
- Use an eye mask for increased relaxation.
- Practice Legs Up the Wall Pose in bed.
- Practice in middle of mat without a wall. Place a block under buttocks and raise straight legs skyward.

VARIATION 1: LEGS ON THE CHAIR POSE

1. Place a chair on the end of the mat. (You may set the chair with its back against the wall for greatest stability.)

2. Begin in Bridge Prep Pose placing your feet in front of the chair.

3. Place your calves and feet up on the chair seat, with or without a blanket under your calves.

4. Your arms can be along your sides, OR in "cactus" position, OR resting on your belly.

5. Lift your heart center toward your chin.

6. Enjoy Legs on the Chair Pose as tolerated, but only 3 to 5 minutes when new to the pose, gradually working up to 20 minutes.

7. To come out of the pose, move slowly, and remain on your side in a fetal position for several breaths.

I have often experienced where my feet were so cold that, regardless if I layered multiple pairs of socks before wrapping my legs under a cozy blanket, any attempt to warm them was futile. Then I learned about Legs Up The Wall Pose. This circulation shift works incredibly well for me! Who knew it could work so fast!

CYNDI, YOGA MOVES STUDENT

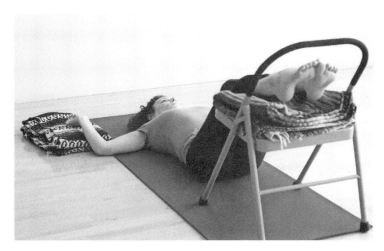

Variation 1: Legs on the Chair Pose

Legs Up the Wall Pose

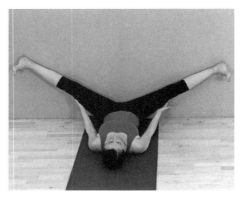

Variation 2: Active Legs Up the Wall Pose with hands on outer thighs

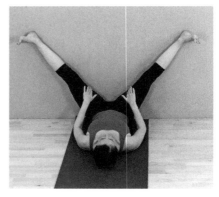

Variation 2: Active Legs Up the Wall Pose with hands on inner thighs

VARIATION 2: ACTIVE LEGS UP THE WALL
INNER THIGH STRENGTHENER WITH RESISTANCE

1. Begin in Legs Up the Wall Pose.
2. Place your hands on the outside of your thighs for support.
3. Open your legs into a "V" against the wall and flex your feet.
4. Move your hands to your inner thighs and press them into your inner thighs, resisting the pressure as you lift the legs. Feel your strength!
5. Repeat Variation 2: Active Legs Up the Wall, alternating opening and lifting your legs for 3 to 5 times.

VARIATION 3: ACTIVE LEGS UP THE WALL
"V" IS FOR VICTORY

1. Flex your feet.
2. Press your right heel into the wall and drag your right leg to the right keeping your left leg skyward.
3. Lift your right leg back to center as you continue to press the heel into the wall.
4. Repeat instructions with your left leg.

5. Open both legs into a "V" pressing both heels against the wall, and then bring them back to center.

6. Repeat sequence of right leg open, left leg open, both legs open, for 1 to 3 times.

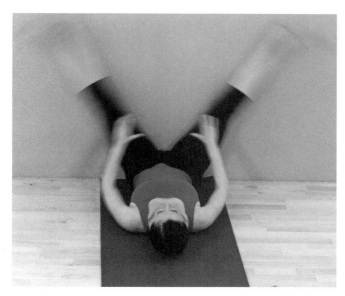

Variation 2 and 3: Active Legs Up the Wall in motion

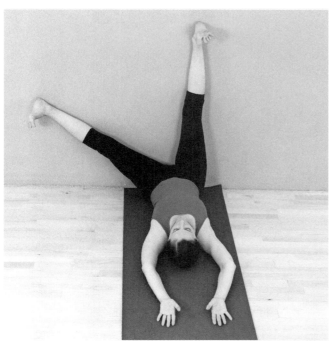

Variation 3: Active Legs Up the Wall with one leg open wide and heel dragging against the wall to build strength

Locust Pose

Salabhasana

PRIMARY BENEFITS

■ Strengthens muscles around the spine

■ Stretches front and back of body

■ Stimulates internal organs

PRECAUTIONS

■ Back or neck condition, injury, or pain

■ Pregnancy

PROPS

■ Yoga mat

■ Blanket

■ Bolster

■ Yoga strap

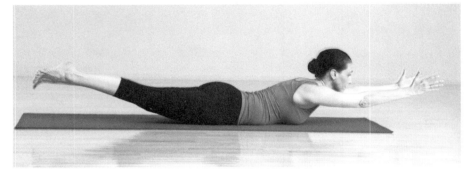

Locust Pose

POSE INSTRUCTIONS

1. Begin on your belly with your forehead on the earth.

2. Lengthen your arms in front of you.

3. Point your toes straight back from your sitting bones. Spread and press them into the mat.

4. Draw your belly in and up as you lengthen your tailbone toward your heels.

5. In a fluid movement, lift your legs, arms, heart center, and shoulders off the mat. Stretch out through your fingers and toes.

6. Lengthen your neck and lift your head, while telescoping your heart forward and up.

7. Keep your gaze forward to your hands, and your heart expanding.

8. Enjoy the Locust Pose for 3 to 5 breaths.

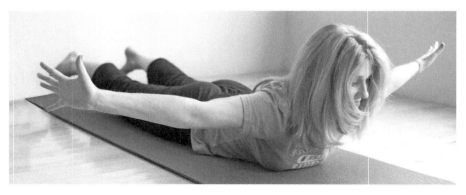

Locust Pose with arms in a "T"

ADAPTATIONS AND VARIATIONS

- Lengthen your arms out to the side in a "T" position.
- Lengthen your arms down by your side, and press the top of your hands into the mat.
- Place your hands under your pelvis for lower back support.
- Lift one leg and the opposite arm. "Karate chop" lower arm into earth. Hold for 3 to 5 breaths. Switch sides.
- Place a rolled blanket or bolster under your chest to support your sternum.
- Place a blanket under your pelvis and rib cage to alleviate pressure.
- Place a strap around shins to keep legs from rolling outward.
- Practice Cobra Pose (see page 156 for instructions).

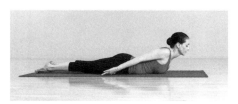

Locust Pose with back of hands pressing down and chest raised

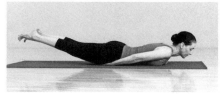

Locust Pose with hands beneath pelvis and both legs raised

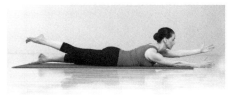

Locust Pose with opposite arm and leg lifted

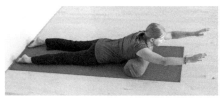

Locust Pose with bolster under chest and arms forward

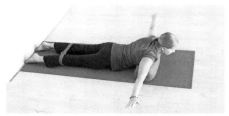

Locust Pose with arms in "T", bolster and strap

Mountain Pose

Tadasana

PRIMARY BENEFITS

- Improves balance and posture
- Increases energy and strength
- Establishes neutral postural alignment in standing position
- Serves as foundation for other standing poses

PRECAUTIONS

- Numbness in feet
- Balance concerns
- Foot, ankle, leg, knee or hip condition, injury, or pain

PROPS

- Yoga mat
- Yoga block
- 1 to 2 Chairs
- Wall

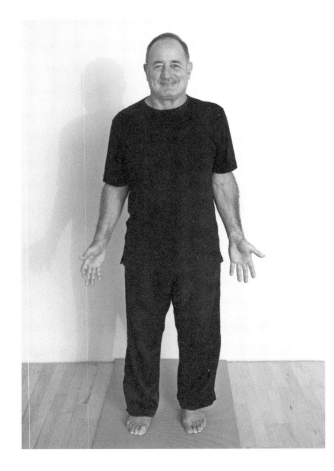

Mountain Pose with palms forward

POSE INSTRUCTIONS

1. Stand tall with your feet, ankles, knees, hips, shoulders, and head aligned from earth to sky. Mountain Pose brings a special awareness to your standing posture.

2. Place your feet hip distance apart, facing forward, and parallel to one another. Check that your toes and knees are pointing forward.

3. Center your weight on your feet, and press them evenly into the earth, with your weight neither too much on the heels, nor on the toes.

4. Stay rooted in your feet as you engage your leg muscles.

5. Create a supported neutral pelvis by lifting your belly in and up as you lengthen your tailbone down.

6. Lengthen your torso by lifting up and out of your waist.

7. Move your shoulders over your hips, drawing the blades together onto your back. With your arms at your sides, open your palms forward. When arms and hands are externally rotated and palms face forward, the shoulders naturally open.

8. Draw the crown of your head skyward while keeping your chin parallel with the earth and your focus forward.

9. Relax your jaw, creating space between your upper and lower teeth. Relax your tongue.

10. Enjoy Mountain Pose for 3 to 5 breaths.

ADAPTATIONS AND VARIATIONS

- Stand in Mountain Pose with back against a wall.
- Stand in Mountain Pose with a chair in front of you and the wall behind you.
- Place a block between your inner thighs or calves.
- Practice Mountain Pose on the Earth. Begin on the earth, drawing special awareness to your posture. Pull your belly in while pressing your head, shoulders, ribs and legs into the earth. Rest your arms by your side, turning palms skyward. Flex your toes and press your heels away from you. Visualize standing in Mountain Pose with your feet pressing into the earth.
- Lift your arm(s) over your head in any of the variations of Mountain Pose.
- Practice Mountain Pose in a Chair (see page 222 for instructions).

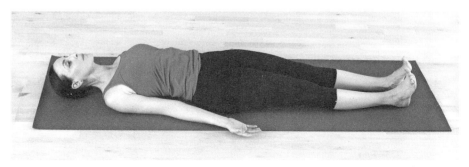

Mountain Pose on the Earth

Mountain Pose in a Chair

Tadasana Variation

PRIMARY BENEFITS

■ Establishes neutral postural alignment

■ Serves as foundation for other seated poses

PRECAUTIONS

■ None known

PROPS

■ Yoga mat

■ Yoga block

■ Yoga strap

■ Towel or extra mat

■ Blanket

■ Chair

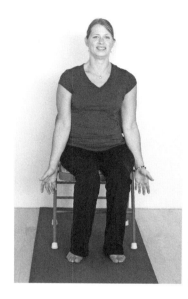

Mountain Pose in a Chair with arms down by side and palms open

POSE INSTRUCTIONS

1. Place a chair on your mat and begin seated on the chair.

2. Place your feet flat on the floor, feeling the soles of your feet touch the earth. Align so that feet are parallel and hip distance apart with knees pointing forward.

3. Establish a neutral spine (not rounded).

4. Stack your shoulders over your hips, and position your head above your shoulders.

5. Establish a neutral lower back curve. Lean into your left hip, place your left hand on your inner right thigh and your right hand on your outer right hip. With the left hand turn the inner thigh muscles down and with the right hand move the flesh outward and back. Repeat on your left side.

6. Feel the weight toward the front of your sitting bones to facilitate a pelvic tilt forward.

7. Lengthen your sitting bones down toward the earth thereby toning your belly for support.

8. With your hands resting on your lap, gently press your palms on your thighs to lift the spine, OR drape arms by your side and face palms forward.

9. Lift your ribs out of your waist and lengthen the sides of your torso.

10. Draw your shoulder blades together onto your back.

11. Draw the crown of your head skyward while keeping your chin parallel with the earth. Sit upright but don't be uptight!

12. Relax your jaw, creating space between your upper and lower teeth. Relax your tongue.

13. Enjoy Mountain Pose in a Chair for 3 to 5 breaths.

ADAPTATIONS AND VARIATIONS

- If your feet do not reach the earth, place a block or blanket under your feet, so the soles of your feet touch a surface.

- Wrap a strap around your thighs for support.

- If your lower back is rounding, try any of the following adaptations: place a rolled towel or mat behind your spine; OR place a cushion, blanket, or towel under your sitting-bones, so your hips are higher than or level with your knees; OR press a block between your inner thighs to feel your midline or center.

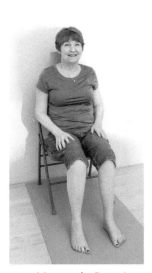

Mountain Pose In a Chair, with rolled mat behind spine

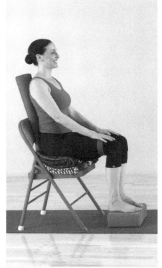

Mountain Pose in a Chair with rolled mat, blanket, yoga blocks, and strap

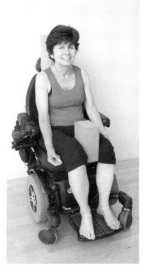

Mountain Pose in a Chair with block and rolled mat

Pelvic Tilt Pose

PRIMARY BENEFITS

■ Warms up and loosens lower back and spine

■ Strengthens abdominal muscles

■ Conditions pelvic floor

PRECAUTIONS

■ Spinal injury

PROPS

■ Yoga mat

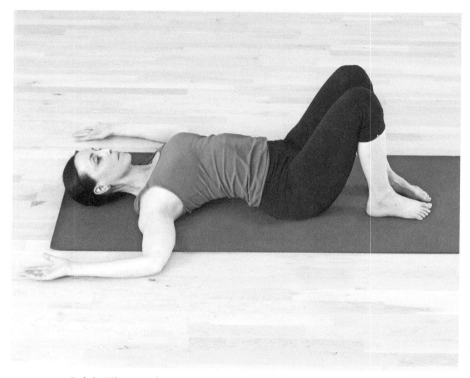

Pelvic Tilt Pose forward with "cactus" arms and upward curve of back

PELVIC TILT POSE FORWARD INSTRUCTIONS

1. Begin in Bridge Prep Pose (see page 137 for instructions).

2. Place your hands on top of your hip bones, OR into "cactus" arms.

3. Tilt the top of pelvis away from the earth and forward so there is space between the back of your waist and the earth. The pubic bone tips down toward the earth while your navel tips skyward.

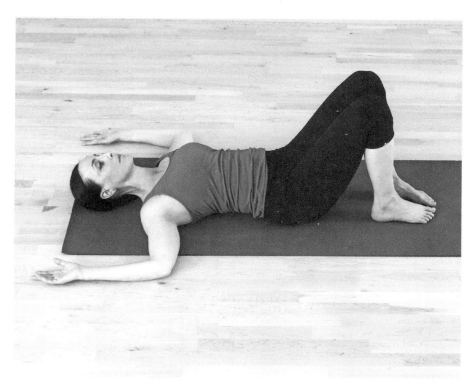

Pelvic Tilt Pose backward with "cactus" arms and back flattened to earth

PELVIC TILT POSE BACKWARD INSTRUCTIONS

1. Keep your hands as in Pelvic Tilt Forward.

2. Tilt the top of the pelvis back toward the earth, so there is no space between the back of your waist and the earth. The pubic bone curls up toward you and your navel pulls in toward the spine.

Pelvic Tilt Pose

COMBINED PELVIC TILT POSE INSTRUCTIONS

1. On your back, tilt your pelvis forward and backward in a rocking motion, releasing the lower back and spine. Match your movements with your breath.

2. The pelvis rocks forward on the inhale and the pelvis rocks backward on the exhale.

3. Repeat a round of Pelvic Tilts 3 to 5 times.

ADAPTATIONS AND VARIATIONS

- To increase the strength of your lower abdominals, contract the navel toward the spine while in Pelvic Tilt Backward. Hold for 3 to 5 counts. Release the contraction completely and return to Pelvic Tilt Forward. Begin with 5 repetitions and increase the number as you become stronger.
- Practice Cat and Cow Poses in a Chair (see page 148 for instructions).
- Practice Cat and Cow Poses (see page 146 for instructions).
- Practice Inchworm Pose (see page 205 for instructions).

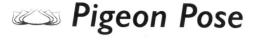 # *Pigeon Pose*

Eka Pada Rajakapotasana

PRIMARY BENEFITS

◼ Opens hips and heart

◼ Stretches groin muscles and thighs

PRECAUTIONS

◼ Spine, psoas muscle, hip, knee, ankle, or foot condition, injury, or pain

PROPS

◼ Yoga mat

◼ Yoga blocks

◼ Blankets

◼ Chair

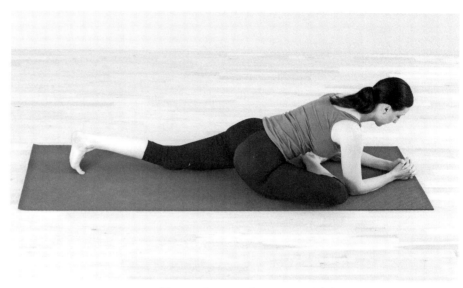

Pigeon Pose on forearms with back toes curled under

POSE INSTRUCTIONS

1. Begin in Table Pose (see page 280 for instructions).

2. Bring your right knee forward between your hands. Widen the knee outward toward your right wrist. Your shin may be at a diagonal with your foot pointing toward your left hip. Press the top of your right foot and toenails into the earth.

3. Extend your left leg back in line with your left sitting bone. Curl the back toes under, OR press the top of the foot and toenails into the earth.

4. Pull your belly in toward your spine.

5. Energetically hug your knees toward each other. Square your hips by pulling your right hip back and your left hip forward. Center your weight equally on both sides. Avoid leaning into your right hip.

6. Stay here or lower onto your forearms.

7. Enjoy Pigeon Pose for 3 to 5 breaths.

8. Practice the instructions above using the opposite side of your body.

Pigeon Pose

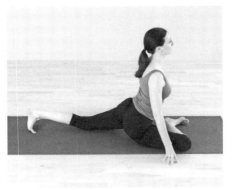 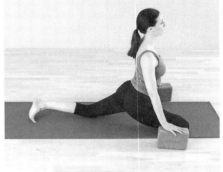

Pigeon Pose upright   Pigeon Pose upright with two blocks

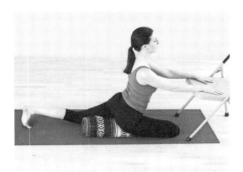

Pigeon Pose with chair and blanket

ADAPTATIONS AND VARIATIONS

- Place a blanket under your back knee for padding.

- Practice upright with hands closer to hips.

- Place both hands on blocks instead of the mat.

- Lengthen your arms forward with your forehead to the earth or on a block.

- Place a blanket or block under your right hip to level both hips.

- Walk your arms to the right and then to the left in a "C" shape for a side stretch on each side.

- Deepen the pose by moving your right shin from its diagonal position to a position more parallel to the front of the mat. Flex your right foot, being careful not to sickle your ankle.

- Practice Pigeon Pose with your hands on the seat of a chair in front of you.

- Practice #4 Pose (see page 130 for instructions).

- Practice Pigeon Pose on your back, known as "Rock the Baby" Pose:

  1. Begin in Bridge Prep Pose (see page 137 for instructions).

  2. Lift your right leg, rotate the knee outward and cradle your right knee and foot between your hands, rocking the leg back and forth as if you were soothing a baby.

  3. If your hips are open and flexible, try placing the flexed right foot in the crook of your left elbow before rocking the baby.

  4. Straighten your bottom left leg for an additional hip stretch.

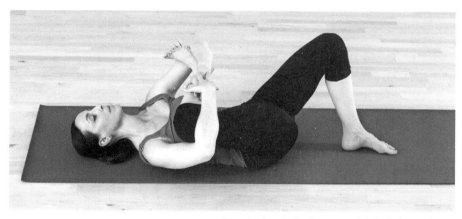

"Rock-the-Baby" Pose with left knee bent

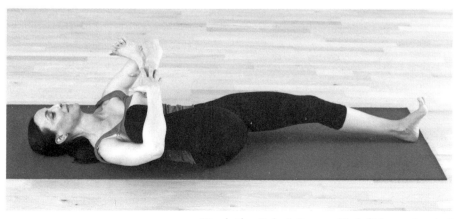

"Rock-the-Baby" Pose, with left leg extended

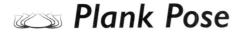

Plank Pose

Chaturanga Variation

PRIMARY BENEFITS

▨ Builds core strength

PRECAUTIONS

▨ Lower back, shoulder, wrist, ankle, or foot condition, injury, or pain

PROPS

▨ Yoga mat

▨ Yoga block

▨ Wall

▨ Yoga dumbells

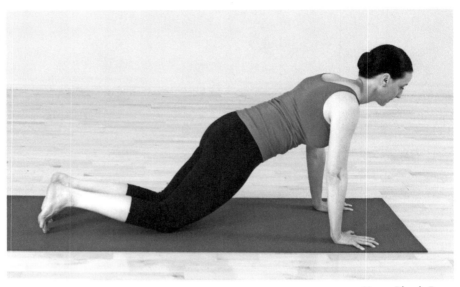

Knee Plank Pose

POSE INSTRUCTIONS

1. Begin in Table Pose (see page 280 for instructions).

2. Walk your knees back as far as you comfortably can while keeping your shoulders over your wrists. Your head, shoulders, hips, and knees will be aligned in a diagonal slope.

3. Spread your fingers and press your hands into the earth, especially the knuckles of your index fingers. This will protect your wrists

4. Draw your belly in and up, and your tailbone down toward your knees. Do not allow the lower back to sag.

5. Draw your shoulder blades together onto your back and hug your forearms toward each other.

6. Gaze forward and down, keeping your neck long. This is called "Knee Plank Pose."

7. For a greater challenge, lift your knees and straighten your legs. Continue to draw your belly in and up and your tailbone down toward your heels. Enjoy Plank Pose for 3 to 5 breaths.

8. Lower into Child's Pose (see page 153 for instructions), OR using your core strength, lift your knees to Downward Facing Dog Pose (see page 170 for instructions).

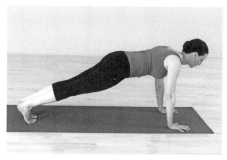

Plank Pose

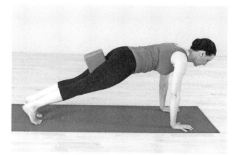

Plank Pose with yoga
block between thighs

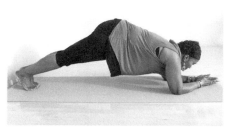

Plank Pose on forearms

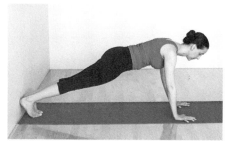

Plank Pose with heels at wall

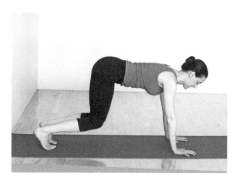

Plank Pose with bent knees lifted off
mat and shoulders over palms

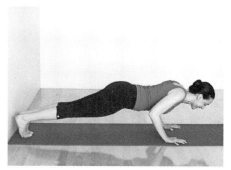

Yoga push-up with heels at wall

Plank Pose

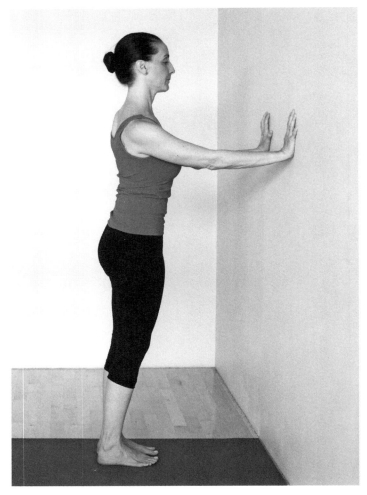

Plank Pose
standing at
the wall

ADAPTATIONS AND VARIATIONS

- Practice with a yoga block between your thighs.
- Practice alternating between raising your knees for Plank Pose and lowering your knees to the earth for Knee Plank Pose.
- Practice Plank Pose or Knee Plank Pose on your forearms.
- Practice Plank Pose from Downward Facing Dog Pose (see page 170 for instructions). Shift your weight forward until your shoulders are over your wrists and your hips are level with your shoulders. You may need to walk your feet back. Draw your belly in and up and your tailbone down toward your heels.

- Practice flowing between Plank Pose and Downward Facing Dog Pose (see page 170 for instructions) 1 to 3 times.

- Practice Plank Pose or Knee Plank Pose with your heels against a wall.

- Practice Plank Pose with bent knees lifted off the mat.

- Practice lowering into a yoga push-up from Plank Pose by bending your elbows and lowering a few inches down, then straightening your arms again. Make sure to keep your shoulders blades together on your back and your elbows close to your body.

- Practice Plank Pose standing at the wall. You may also practice a yoga push-up at the wall, with or without yoga dumbbells.

- Practice Table Pose (see page 280 for instructions) on your forearms.

Adaptive yoga gives me a way to communicate with my mind, body and soul.

DON, YOGA MOVES STUDENT

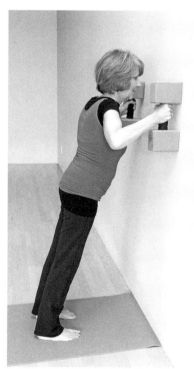

Push-up at wall with yoga dumbbells: into wall

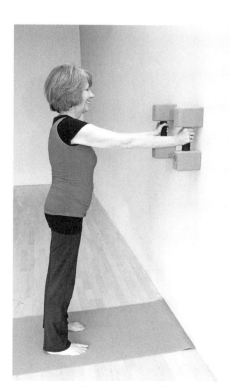

Push-up at wall with yoga dumbbells: away from wall

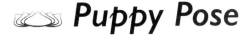 # *Puppy Pose*

Anahatasana

PRIMARY BENEFITS

■ Opens shoulder girdle

■ Lengthens spine and arms

PRECAUTIONS

■ Shoulder, spine, or knee condition, injury, or pain

PROPS

■ Yoga mat

■ Yoga block

■ Blanket

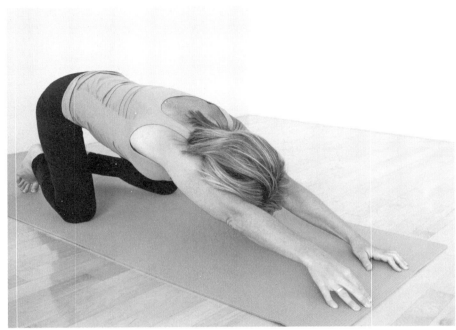

Puppy Pose

POSE INSTRUCTIONS

1. Begin in Table Pose (see page 280 for instructions).

2. Walk your hands forward as your arms lengthen and your heart lowers toward the earth. Keep your hips over your knees. Your chin or forehead may rest on the earth.

3. Press your hands into the earth to lift the underside of your arms and pull your shoulder blades together onto your back.

4. Lengthen your tailbone down to your knees, and pull your belly in and up.

5. Enjoy Puppy Pose for 3 to 5 breaths.

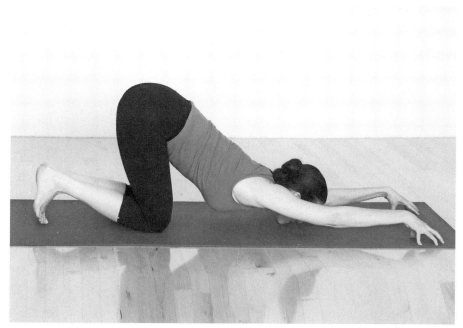

Puppy Pose with "spider" hands

ADAPTATIONS AND VARIATIONS

- Place a blanket or block under your forehead to elevate your head.
- Place a folded blanket under your knees.
- Press your fingertips into the mat for "spider" hands.
- Practice Child's Pose (see page 153 for instructions).

Pyramid Pose

Parsvottanasana

PRIMARY BENEFITS

■ Lengthens spine, arms, and legs

■ Opens hips

■ Strengthens lower body

■ Improves balance

PRECAUTIONS

■ Balance concerns

■ Spine, hip, knee, or ankle condition, injury, or pain

PROPS

■ Yoga mat

■ Yoga blocks

■ Chair

■ Wall

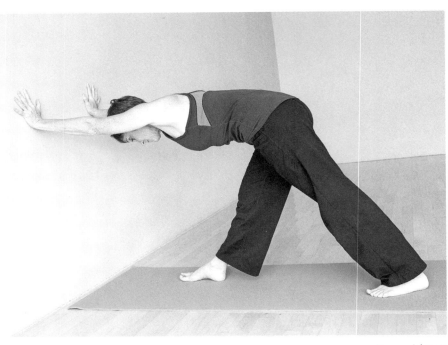

Pyramid Pose

POSE INSTRUCTIONS

1. Begin in Mountain Pose facing the wall (see page 220 for instructions).
2. Place your hands on the wall at shoulder height and shoulder distance apart.
3. Walk backward and bend at the hips until your body begins to look like an "L" with your arms outstretched.
4. Step your right foot forward with your toes facing the wall. The distance is based on your current flexibility and balance.
5. Turn your left foot to the left about 45 degrees away from your body. Your legs should be about hip width apart.
6. Keep both legs straight. Maintain a micro bend in your knees to avoid hyperextension.
7. Adjust your stance: the width of your stance will increase the stability in the pose; and the length of your stance will increase the intensity of the stretch.

8. Square your hips to the wall by moving your right hip back and your left hip forward.

9. Press your feet firmly into the earth, and hug them toward each other, OR press them away from each other to feel your strength.

10. Lift up out of your waist and extend your crown forward toward the wall. Gazing toward the earth, keep your ears level with your arms.

11. Enjoy Pyramid Pose for 3 to 5 breaths.

12. Practice the instructions above using the opposite side of your body.

ADAPTATIONS AND VARIATIONS

• Place your hands on a chair placed against a wall for more stability.

• Practice the pose in the middle of your mat. Place your hands on the earth, OR use blocks to "raise the earth" to your hands.

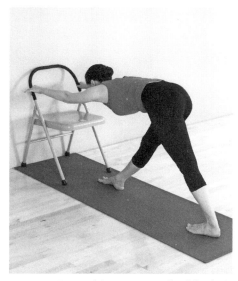

Pyramid Pose at wall with chair

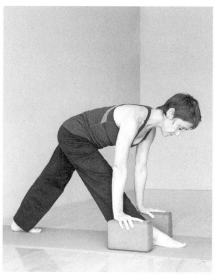

Pyramid Pose in the middle of mat with blocks

Relaxation Pose

Savasana

PRIMARY BENEFITS

■ Provides time to absorb benefits of a yoga practice

■ Relaxes and rejuvenates body and mind

■ Calms central nervous system, reducing stress and anxiety

PRECAUTIONS

■ Spinal condition, injury, or pain

■ Pregnancy

PROPS

■ Yoga mat

■ Yoga strap

■ Blankets

■ Sandbags

■ Eye cover

■ Small towel or washcloth

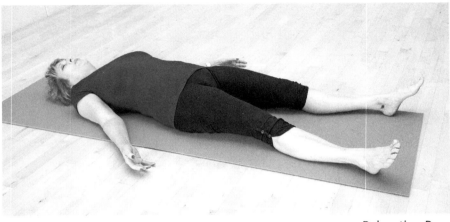

Relaxation Pose

POSE INSTRUCTIONS

1. Begin in Mountain Pose on the earth (see page 221 for instructions).

2. Angle your heels toward the corners of your mat and allow your feet to open out to the side naturally.

3. Close your eyes and cover them with an eye mask or a washcloth if desired.

4. With your arms at your sides, open your palms skyward, in a receptive mode. When the arms and hands are externally rotated and palms face upward, the shoulders naturally open.

5. Soften your jaw, the root of your tongue, and your forehead.

6. Allow your eyes to feel heavy in their sockets, and draw your inner gaze toward your heart.

7. Enjoy Relaxation Pose for 3 to 20 minutes, focusing on your natural breath.

8. To come out of the pose, lift your right arm overhead and behind you. Roll to your right side into a fetal position, with your head resting on your right arm. Remain in fetal position for a few breaths, before using your hands to help you rise to a seated position. Remain seated in Easy Pose (see page 175 for instructions) for several breaths to express gratitude for your practice and re-enter your day refreshed.

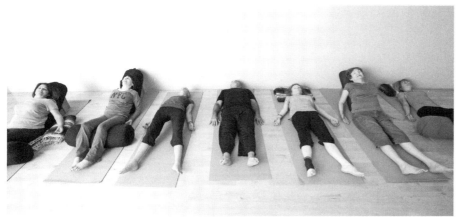

Relaxation Pose, a well deserved rest after a rewarding yoga practice

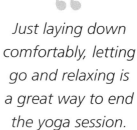

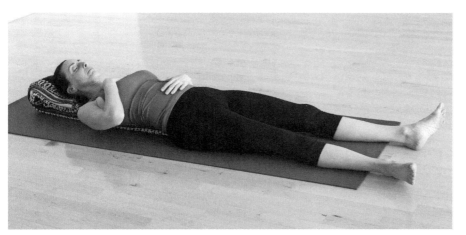

Relaxation Pose with folded blanket under neck and head

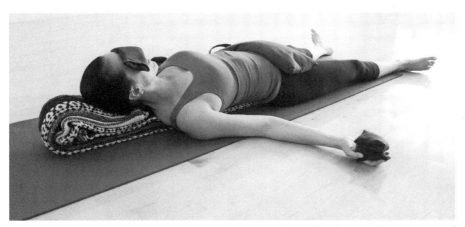

Relaxation Pose with sandbags on belly and palms, and eyes covered

Relaxation Pose

ADAPTATIONS AND VARIATIONS

- Cover yourself with a blanket if desired.
- Place one hand on your heart and the other on your belly, OR both hands on your belly.
- Place a folded blanket under your head OR a rolled cloth under your neck.
- Play soothing music while in Relaxation Pose.
- Use a bolster propped with blocks OR blankets under the torso for a heart opening Relaxation Pose.
- Place a bolster or rolled blanket under your knees
- Pad the mat with extra blankets for comfort.
- Practice Relaxation Pose in a chair. Sit quietly in a chair with your eyes closed and hands on thighs OR in lap. Relax your body and your mind.
- Practice Relaxation Pose with two chairs. Use one chair for your seat and the other chair for your legs.
- Practice Legs Up the Wall (see page 212 for instructions).
- Practice Restorative Butterfly Pose (see page 245 for instructions).

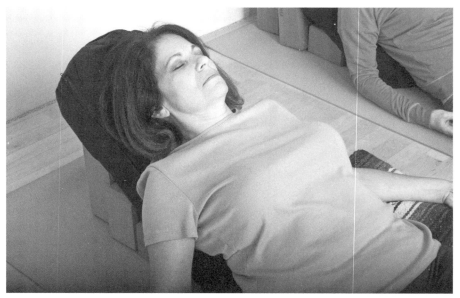

Deep Relaxation Pose with bolster, blocks and blankets

Restorative Backbend Poses

Setu Bandha Sarvangasana Variation

PRIMARY BENEFITS

■ Opens front of body

■ Improves posture

■ Increases energy

■ Reduces fatigue, low back pain, and leg swelling

PRECAUTIONS

■ Eye problems, including glaucoma

■ Neck, shoulder, or spinal condition, injury, or pain

■ Pregnant over three months, or menstruating

PROPS

■ Yoga mat

■ Yoga blocks

■ Yoga strap

■ Blankets

■ 2 bolsters

■ Small towel or washcloth

■ Sandbags

■ Eye cover

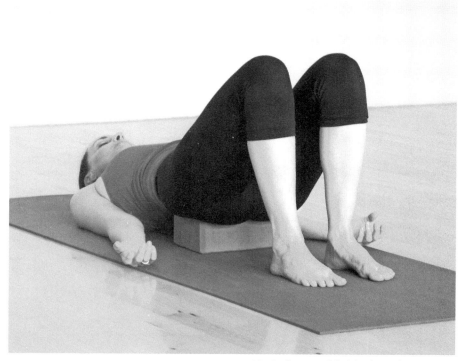

Variation 1 with block under sacrum

POSE INSTRUCTIONS

VARIATION 1

1. Begin in Bridge Prep Pose (see page 137 for instructions).

2. Place a yoga block, OR a tightly folded blanket, under your hips. Find just the right spot so that you feel comfortable in the pose.

3. Enjoy Variation 1 for 3 to 5 minutes initially, and gradually work up to longer increments if desired.

4. To exit the pose, slowly bring your knees into your chest, and roll to your right side for a few breaths.

Restorative Backbend Poses

VARIATION 2

1. Begin in Bridge Prep Pose (see page 137 for instructions).

2. Place a tightly rolled blanket horizontally under the tips of shoulders blades. Find just the right spot so that you feel comfortable in the pose.

3. Place your arms in "cactus" or "T" position, with palms facing skyward.

4. Enjoy Variation 2 for 3 to 5 minutes initially, and gradually work up to longer increments if desired.

5. To exit the pose, slowly bring your knees into your chest, and roll to your right side for a few breaths.

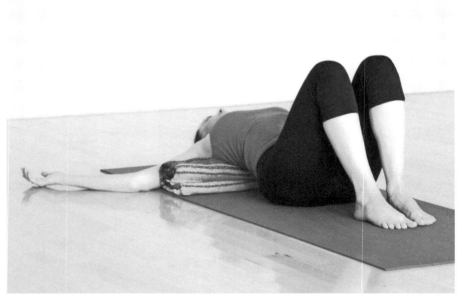

Variation 2 with rolled blanket under shoulder blades

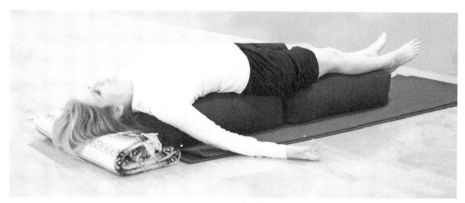

Variation 3 with two bolsters and blanket

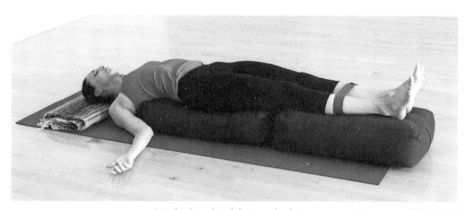

Variation 3 with two bolsters, yoga strap, and blanket

VARIATION 3

1. Place 2 bolsters end to end along the length of your mat, and a folded blanket at one end for your head.

2. Recline onto the bolsters. Your arms, shoulders, neck, and head should gently drape off the bolster onto the earth.

3. You may place a yoga strap around your ankles for additional support.

4. Turn your palms skyward.

5. Relax and breathe as you feel the support of the earth and props.

6. Enjoy Variation 3 for 3 to 5 minutes initially and gradually work up to longer increments if desired.

7. To exit the pose, slowly bring your knees into your chest, and roll off the bolster onto your right side for a few breaths.

Restorative Backbend Poses

VARIATION 4

1. Place a bolster under your hips and upper thighs.

2. Place a folded blanket under your feet.

3. Place a rolled blanket horizontally underneath your shoulder blades.

4. Proper head and neck alignment is important. Experiment with a blanket under your head or a rolled towel under your neck to support a natural curve.

5. Position your arms in a "T" or in "cactus" arms.

6. Enjoy Variation 4 for 3 to 5 minutes initially and gradually work up to longer increments if desired.

7. To exit the pose, slowly bring your knees into your chest, and roll off the bolster onto your right side for a few breaths.

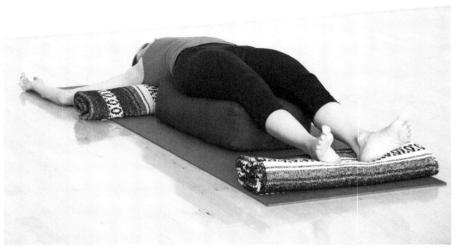

Variation 4 with bolster under hips and legs, rolled blankets under shoulders, and folded blanket under feet

Restorative Butterfly Pose

Baddha Konasana Variation

PRIMARY BENEFITS

■ Opens heart center and shoulders

■ Relaxes and refreshes nervous system and reduces fatigue

■ Stretches inner thighs and increases hip flexibility

■ Increases circulation to digestive organs

PRECAUTIONS

■ Spinal, hip, or knee pain, injury, or condition

■ Pregnancy

PROPS

■ Yoga mat

■ Yoga block

■ Yoga strap

■ Bolster

■ Blankets

■ Sandbags for eyes, palms, or belly

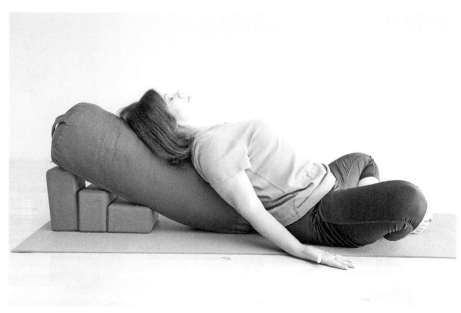

Restorative Butterfly Pose

POSE INSTRUCTIONS

1. Place a bolster lengthwise at the top of your mat. Insert 1 to 3 yoga blocks under the top of the bolster to angle the bolster into an incline that suits your comfort and preferences.

2. Sit with your back facing the lower end of the bolster.

3. Bend your knees and open them to your sides. Bring the soles of your feet together, forming a "butterfly".

4. Support your knees and outer thighs with a block or rolled blanket under them.

5. Lie back onto the bolster.

6. Open your arms to your sides, with your palms facing skyward.

7. For greater comfort and relaxation, you may wish to place blankets under your arms and hands; place weighted bags on your palms, especially if you hold tension in your fingers and hands; place a mask over your eyes; and place a weighted bag on your belly.

Restorative Butterfly Pose

8. Enjoy the Restorative Butterfly Pose for 3 to 5 minutes initially, and gradually work up to longer increments.

9. To exit the pose, roll to your right into a fetal position for a few breaths, then rise carefully and sit in Easy Pose for 3 to 5 breaths (see page 175 for instructions).

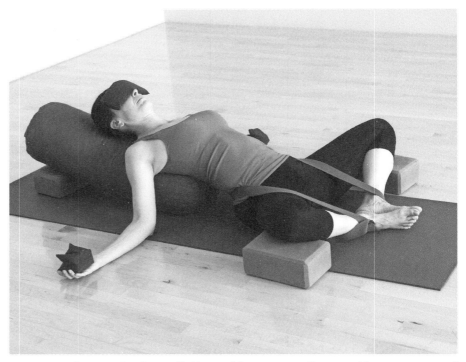

Restorative Butterfly Pose with strap, sandbags and knees supported

ADAPTATIONS AND VARIATIONS

- Support your knees and thighs with blocks OR rolled blankets.

- Use a rolled blanket in lieu of the bolster under your spine.

- Practice Restorative Butterfly Pose with a yoga strap supporting your legs and hips. Begin by wrapping a strap around your lower back. Bring ends forward over your hips and across your thighs. Next, wrap strap over your ankles and under the outside edge of your feet. Cinch or buckle the strap.

Restorative Forward Fold Pose

Salamba Paschimottanasana

PRIMARY BENEFITS

■ Encourages inner focus

■ Calms nervous system

■ Aids digestion

■ Neutralizes backbends

PRECAUTIONS

■ Spine or neck condition, injury, or pain

PROPS

■ Yoga mat

■ Yoga strap

■ Blankets

■ Chair

■ Bolster

■ Table

Restorative Forward Fold Pose over chair with blanket and straight arms

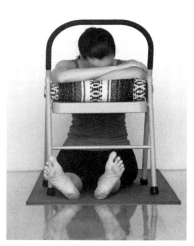

Restorative Forward Fold Pose over chair with blanket and folded arms

POSE INSTRUCTIONS

1. Place a chair at one end of your mat.

2. Sit on the earth in front of the chair.

3. Slide your legs under the chair, extending them as in Stick Pose (see page 276 for instructions).

4. Fold your arms over the seat of the chair, OR lay them straight across chair.

5. Rest your forehead on your forearms, OR turn your head to the side. If you do turn your head, make sure to spend equal amounts of time on each side.

6. Make adjustments for your comfort and ease.

7. Enjoy the Restorative Forward Fold Pose for 3 to 5 minutes initially, and gradually work up to longer increments if desired.

8. To exit the pose, place your hands on the chair to slowly sit up, OR place them behind you to help support your weight, as you slowly come out of the pose.

Restorative Forward Fold Pose

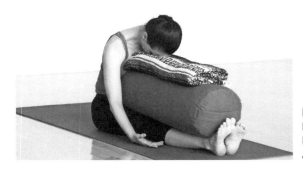

Restorative Forward Fold Pose over blanket and bolster

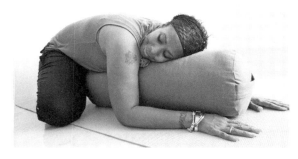

Child's Pose with bolster

ADAPTATIONS AND VARIATIONS

- Place blankets under your hips to support the natural curve of your lower spine.

- Stack blankets on the seat of the chair to support your arms, neck, head, and spine.

- Practice Restorative Forward Fold Pose over a bolster. Begin in Stick Pose (see page 276 for instructions). Stack a bolster and blanket on top of your legs. Rest your forehead on stack and let your arms drape down by your side. Adjust the angle of your spine with more blankets on the bolster so that there is no strain in your neck or spine and to encourage relaxation.

- Practice Restorative Forward Fold Pose in a chair. Stack your forearms on a table in front of you, and rest your forehead on your arms.

- Practice Child's Pose with a bolster (see page 153 for instructions).

- Practice Forward Fold Pose (see page 182 for instructions).

- Practice Restorative Wide Angle Forward Fold (see page 317 for instructions).

Restorative Twist Pose Over Bolster

Salamba Jathara Parivartanasana

PRIMARY BENEFITS

■ Stretches sides of the body and muscles between ribs

■ Increases breath flow

■ Relieves back pain

■ Improves digestion

PRECAUTIONS

■ Spinal condition, injury, or pain

PROPS

■ Yoga mat

■ Blankets

■ Bolster

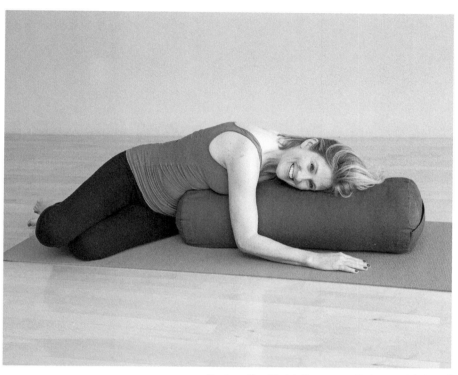

Restorative Twist Pose over Bolster with head in the same direction as knees

POSE INSTRUCTIONS

1. Place a bolster lengthwise on your mat.

2. Begin seated with your right hip next to the bottom of the bolster and your knees bent.

3. Gently twist your torso and lower your chest onto the bolster.

4. Turn your head to either side. For a more complete twist, the head twists in the opposite direction of the knees.

5. Allow your arms to gently drape over the sides of the bolster.

6. Enjoy the Restorative Twist Pose over Bolster for 1 to 3 minutes initially and gradually work up to longer increments.

7. Practice the instructions above using the opposite side of your body.

Restorative Twist Pose Over Bolster

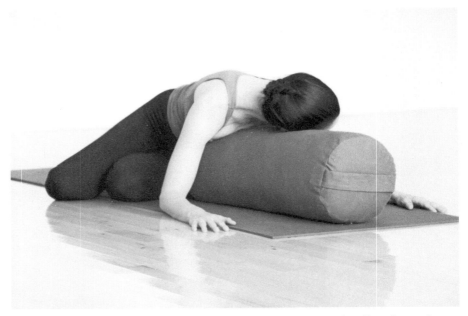

Restorative Twist Pose over Bolster with head in opposite direction as knees

ADAPTATIONS AND VARIATIONS

- Use a stack of folded blankets instead of a bolster.
- Practice Spinal Twist Pose Reclining (see page 274 for instructions).

Reverse Triangle Pose

Parivrtta Trikonasana

PRIMARY BENEFITS

- Lengthens legs, arms, and spine

- Energizes body

- Strengthens legs and core

- Improves digestion

- Reduces piriformis syndrome and sciatica

- Opens heart, shoulders and hips

PRECAUTIONS

- Balance concerns

- Spine or hip condition, injury, or pain

PROPS

- Yoga mat
- Yoga block
- Chair
- Wall

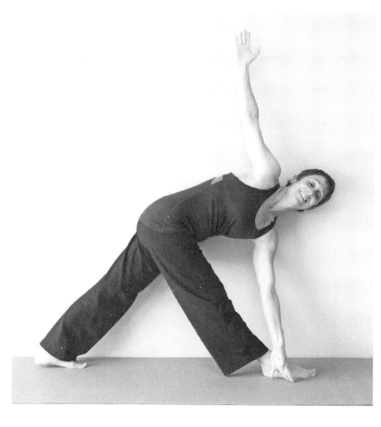

Reverse Triangle Pose with arm raised

POSE INSTRUCTIONS

1. Place the long side of your mat against the wall.
2. Stand in the middle of the mat with your left hip against the wall.
3. Step your right foot forward.
4. Square your hips by moving the outside of your right hip backward and the outside of your left hip forward.
5. Place your right hand on your right hip. Raise your left arm overhead to lift long through your spine. Pull your belly in and up.
6. Hinge at the hips, and reach forward and down. Place your left hand on the earth either inside or outside your right foot.
7. Lengthen your torso as you lean into the wall and extend your tailbone down.

Reverse Triangle Pose

8. Begin to twist from your navel and then continue the twist up your spine as your heart opens away from the wall.

9. Reach your right hand skyward to deepen the twist.

10. Gaze toward your right toes, OR forward, OR to your raised right hand.

11. Enjoy Reverse Triangle Pose for 3 to 5 breaths.

12. Practice the instructions above using the opposite side of your body.

ADAPTATIONS AND VARIATIONS

- If your left hand does not reach the earth, use a block to raise the earth to your hand, OR prop your left hand on a chair placed in front of you.

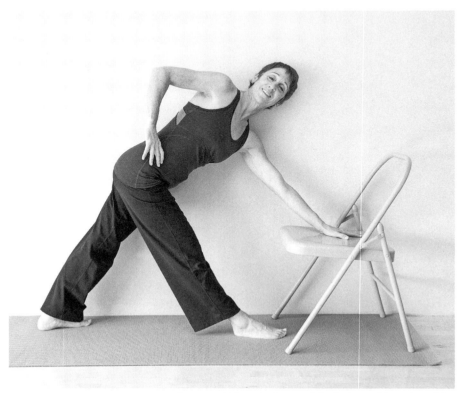

Reverse Triangle Pose with chair and hand on hip

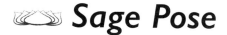 # Sage Pose

Marichyasana A

PRIMARY BENEFITS

■ Lengthens spine

■ Strengthens core

■ Opens shoulders

■ Stimulates bottom of feet

PRECAUTIONS

■ Spine or back, knee, or foot condition, injury, or pain

PROPS

■ Yoga mat

■ Yoga strap

■ 2 chairs

■ Blankets

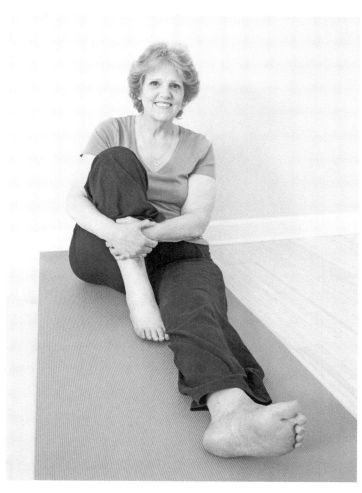

Sage Pose

POSE INSTRUCTIONS

1. Begin in Stick Pose (see page 276 for instructions).
2. Lift your right knee and place the foot on the earth in front of your right sitting bone.
3. Press your left thigh and your right foot into the earth.
4. Place your hands around the front of your right shin, and pull inward as you lift your heart.
5. Enjoy Sage Pose for 3 to 5 breaths.
6. Practice the instructions above using the opposite side of your body.

Sage Pose

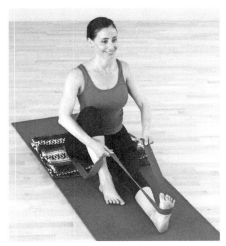

Sage Pose with yoga strap and blanket

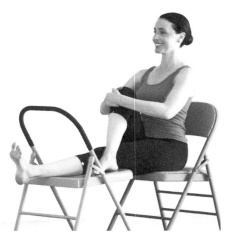

Sage Pose with two chairs, with right foot outside left knee

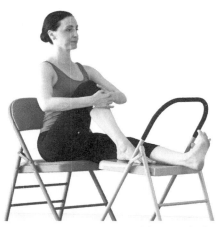

Sage Pose with two chairs

ADAPTATIONS AND VARIATIONS

- Place a cushion, blanket, or towel under your sitting bones so that your lower spine is neutral (not rounded).
- Practice Sage Pose on two chairs facing each other.
- Place a yoga strap around your left foot and pull gently toward you as you lift your heart.
- Place a folded blanket or rolled mat under your left knee to prevent it from locking.
- Place your right foot outside your left knee.

Sage Twist Pose

Marichyasana C

PRIMARY BENEFITS

■ Lengthens spine

■ Strengthens core

■ Opens shoulders

■ Stimulates bottom
of feet

■ Improves digestion

PRECAUTIONS

■ Spine or back
condition, injury, or pain

PROPS

■ Yoga mat

■ 2 chairs

■ Blankets

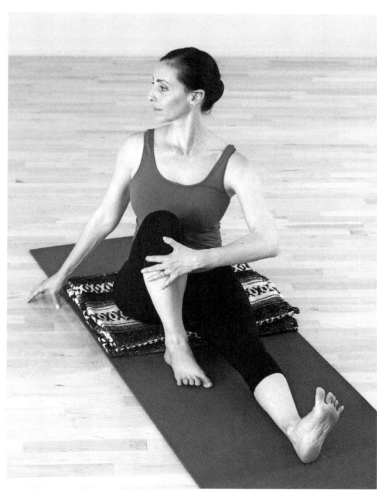

Sage Twist
Pose

POSE INSTRUCTIONS

1. Begin in Stick Pose (see page 276 for instructions).
2. Lift your right knee and place the foot flat on the earth in front of your right hip.
3. Press your left thigh into the earth.
4. Place your hands around the front of the right shin while you press your right foot down and lift your heart.
5. Draw your lower belly in and up.

Sage Twist Pose

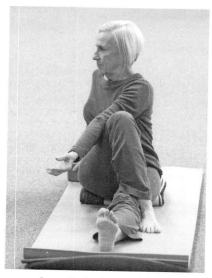

Sage Twist Pose with right leg crossed outside left knee

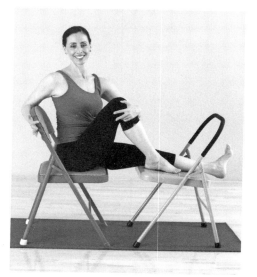

Sage Twist Pose in two chairs

6. Begin to twist to the right from your navel, place your right hand behind you, and continue the twist up your spine.

7. Roll your right shoulder back.

8. Turn your head toward the right after you have twisted your spine. Be careful not to strain your neck by turning your head too far to the right.

9. Enjoy Sage Twist Pose for 3 to 5 breaths.

10. Practice the instructions above using the opposite side of your body.

ADAPTATIONS AND VARIATIONS

- Place a blanket under your sitting bones so that your lower spine is neutral (not rounded).
- Place a folded blanket or rolled mat under your left knee to prevent it from locking.
- Use your left hand to pull your right leg to the left to find a deeper twist.
- Place your left elbow outside your right knee.
- Cross your right foot outside your left knee as you twist to the right.
- Practice Sage Twist Pose on two chairs, extending your left leg and placing your right foot on the chair in front of you.
- Practice Sage Twist Pose in a chair. Sit on the edge of the chair. Extend your left leg long and press the heel into the earth. You may place a block under your right foot. Place your forearm on the outside of the right thigh. Place your right hand on the back of the chair and twist to the right.

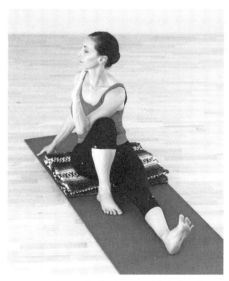

Sage Twist Pose with left elbow
outside of right knee

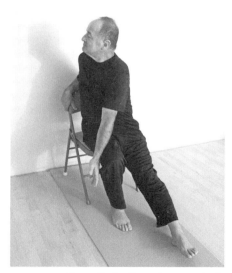

Sage Twist Pose in one chair

Scale Pose

Tolasana

PRIMARY BENEFITS

■ Builds core and upper body strength

PRECAUTIONS

■ Shoulder, elbow, wrist, hip, knee, or ankle condition, injury, or pain

PROPS

■ Yoga mat

■ Yoga blocks

■ Chair

■ Blanket

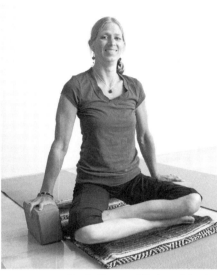

Scale Pose with two blocks

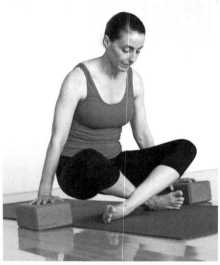

Scale Pose with hands pressing into two blocks

POSE INSTRUCTIONS

1. Begin in Easy Pose (see page 175 for instructions).

2. Place blocks by your hips and rest your hands on them.

3. Exhale, pull your belly in and up. Press your palms into the blocks and lift your hips, and possibly your feet, off the earth.

4. Inhale and return your hips to the earth.

5. Repeat Scale Pose 3 to 5 times.

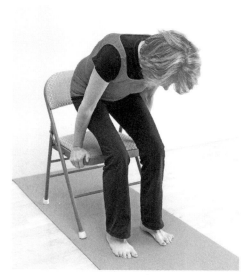

Scale Pose in a chair

ADAPTATIONS AND VARIATIONS

- Sit on a blanket for comfort.

- Practice Scale Pose seated in a chair. Place your hands on the side of the seat and look toward your belly as you pull it in and up. Press down with your hands and lift your hips on the exhale. Relax your hands and place hips down on the chair on the inhale.

- To increase the height of your lift while seated on the earth, turn the blocks on their sides, cupping your hands over the top of the blocks to provide additional stability.

- Practice Scale Pose with your hands on the earth rather than on blocks.

Side Plank Pose

Vasisthasana Variation

PRIMARY BENEFITS

■ Builds core strength

■ Tones and lengthens sides of body

■ Builds upper body strength

■ Improves balance

■ Lessens effects of scoliosis

PRECAUTIONS

■ Neck, shoulder, elbow, wrist, hip, knee, ankle condition, injury, or pain

PROPS

■ Yoga mat

■ Yoga block

■ Chair

■ Wall

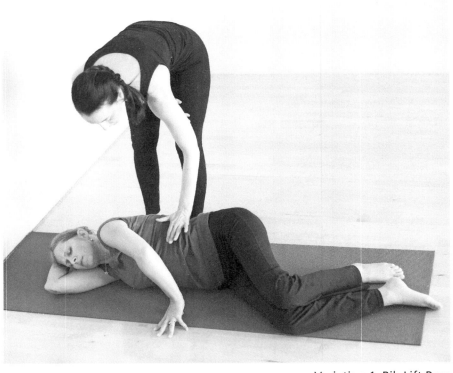

Variation 1: Rib Lift Pose

POSE INSTRUCTIONS
VARIATION 1: RIB LIFT POSE

1. Begin by lying on your right side on the earth.

2. Bend your knees for stability, and place your right arm under your head for support, with your elbow bent, OR with your right arm stretched long.

3. Place your left hand on the earth in front of your torso for stability.

4. Keeping your right hip and shoulder on the earth, exhale and lift your lower ribs up off of the earth. This is a very subtle movement and not easy to see but you can feel it.

5. Inhale and lower your ribs.

6. Enjoy Variation 1: Rib Lift 5 to 10 times.

7. Practice the instructions above using the opposite side of your body.

HAND PLACEMENT INSTRUCTIONS FOR VARIATIONS 2 THROUGH 5

Correct shoulder placement is very important. For Pose Variations 2 through 5, place your right hand on the earth toward the top of the mat, slightly forward of your shoulder and in line with your hip. Protect your right shoulder by angling your right fingers to the right and point your fingers toward one o'clock. This will help your shoulder blades move together on your back and toward your spine. It will also help you rotate the arm and shoulder toward the right.

There are two positions that should be avoided for proper shoulder health: when the right shoulder projects beyond your wrists toward the top of the mat; and when the right shoulder rolls forward toward the side of your mat. Please refrain from either of these shoulder positions.

VARIATION 2: HALF PLANK POSE

1. Begin on the earth sitting on your right hip, with both knees bent and stacked.

2. Place your right hand on the earth as indicated with instructions above. Place your left hand on your left hip. Alternative left hand placements can include placing your left hand on the earth, OR a block, OR a chair in front of you.

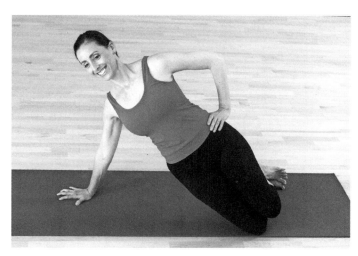

Variation 2:
Half Plank Pose,
hips lifted

Side Plank Pose

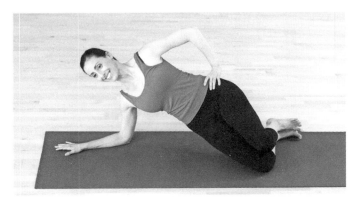

Variation 2: Half Plank Pose on forearm, hips lifted

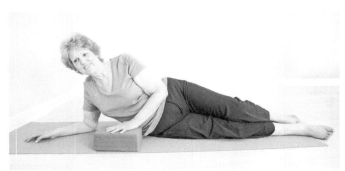

Variation 2: Half Plank Pose with hips on earth, resting on forearm and block

3. Draw your shoulder blades together onto your back.

4. Spread your right fingers and press into the earth through the base of the index finger.

5. Press down through your right hand as you lift your hips and torso. Your knees stay grounded. Your body will be on a diagonal from your right shoulder to your right knee. Be conscious of the position of your right shoulder. Lower down to adjust your hand placement if necessary.

6. Enjoy Variation 2: Half Plank Pose for 3 to 5 breaths.

7. You may also raise your left hand skyward, or extend it over your left ear to feel a stretch along your entire left side.

8. Practice the instructions above using the opposite side of your body.

Adaptations of Variation 2 can include practicing the pose on your right forearm with hips raised OR on the earth.

VARIATION 3: GATE POSE

Parighasana

1. Begin in Table Pose (see page 280 for instructions).

2. Place your right hand on the earth, as indicated in instructions above. Place your left hand on your left hip. Alternative left hand placements can include placing your left hand on the earth, OR a block, OR a chair in front of you.

3. Extend your left leg back and place the inside edge of your left foot on the mat. Your right knee remains on the earth. Swing your right lower leg to the right, so that it is almost parallel with the short end of your mat. Curl your right toes under.

4. Press into your left foot and right hand to open your torso to the left.

5. Roll your shoulder blades together onto your back and turn your heart skyward.

6. Enjoy Variation 3: Gate Pose for 3 to 5 breaths.

7. Practice the instructions above using the opposite side of your body.

Adaptation for Variation 3 can include practicing the pose on your right forearm; raising your left arm skyward, OR extending your left arm over your left ear.

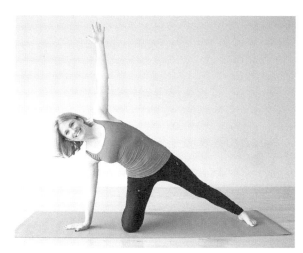

Variation 3:
Gate Pose

Side Plank Pose

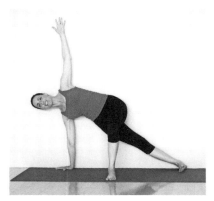

Variation 4: Side Plank Pose with "Kickstand"and arm skyward at wall

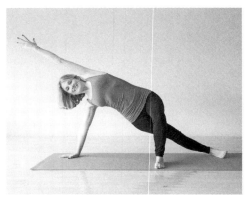

Variation 4: Side Plank Pose with "Kickstand" with arm over ear

VARIATION 4: SIDE PLANK POSE WITH "KICKSTAND"

1. Begin on the earth sitting on your right hip with both knees bent and stacked.

2. Place your right hand on the earth as indicated with instructions above. Place your left hand or your left hip. Alternative left hand placements include on the earth, OR a block, OR a chair in front of you.

3. Draw your shoulder blades together on your back. Spread your right fingers and press into the earth through the pointer finger knuckle.

4. Place your left foot on the earth in front of your right hip as a "kickstand."

5. Straighten your right leg toward the back of the mat.

6. Press down through your right hand, your left foot, and the outside edge of your right foot, to lift your hips. Experiment with the placement of your left foot to maximize leverage and support.

7. When you lift your hips, be concious of the position of your right shoulder. Lower down and adjust your hand placement if necessary.

8. For support, lean your head, shoulders and hips against a wall.

9. Enjoy Variation 4: Side Plank Pose with "Kickstand" for 3 to 5 breaths.

10. Practice the instructions above using the opposite side of your body.

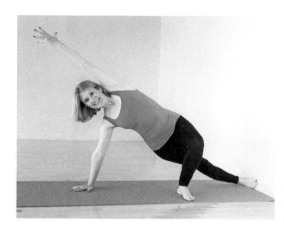

Variation 5: Side Plank Pose with "Kickstand" and Foot at Wall

VARIATION 5: SIDE PLANK POSE WITH "KICKSTAND" AND FOOT AT WALL

1. Place your mat with the short edge against the wall.

2. Follow all instructions for Variation 4 except place your bottom foot against the wall.

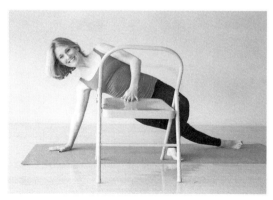

Variation 4: Side Plank Pose with "Kickstand" and chair

ADAPTATIONS TO VARIATIONS 4 AND 5

- Practice with a chair in front of you for support.
- Practice on your forearm instead of your hand.

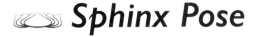 # Sphinx Pose

Salamba Bhujangasana

PRIMARY BENEFITS

■ Opens shoulders and heart center

■ Lengthens front of body

■ Strengthens upper body

■ Stimulates digestive organs

PRECAUTIONS

■ Lower back, shoulder, or neck condition, injury, or pain.

■ Pregnancy

PROPS

■ Yoga mat

■ Yoga block

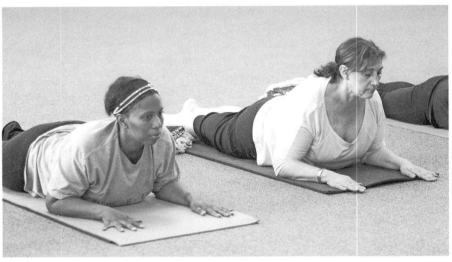

Sphinx Pose

POSE INSTRUCTIONS

1. Begin on your belly.

2. Place your forearms in front of you, parallel to one another, with your elbows bent and under your shoulders.

3. Point your toes straight back from your sitting bones. Spread and press them into the mat.

4. Draw your belly in and up as you lengthen your tailbone toward your heels.

5. Press down on your forearms and energetically pull your elbows, forearms and hands toward your hips.

6. In a fluid movement, lift your chest and shoulders off the mat, and roll your shoulder blades together onto your back.

7. Lengthen your neck and lift your head, while telescoping your heart forward and up.

8. Keep your gaze forward and your heart expanding.

9. Enjoy Sphinx Pose for 3 to 5 breaths.

ADAPTATIONS AND VARIATIONS

- With hands forming an "L" shape, place the corners of a block between your thumb and forefingers. Press into the block.

- Practice Sphinx Pose in a chair at the wall. Refer to Cobra Pose in a Chair at the Wall for pose preparation (see page 158 for instructions), placing elbows onto wall at shoulder height.

- Practice Sphinx Pose while standing facing a wall.

- Practice Sphinx Pose Core Builder (see page 94 for instructions).

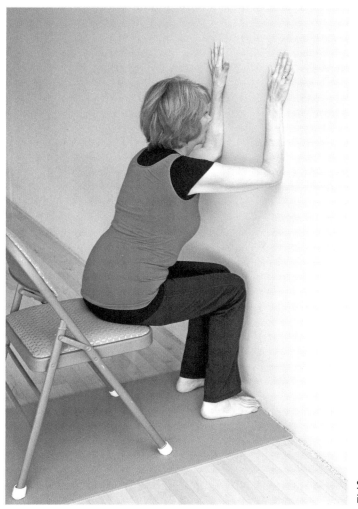

Sphinx Pose
in chair

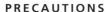 # Spinal Balance Pose

PRIMARY BENEFITS

▓ Improves balance, focus, and coordination

▓ Strengthens body, especially muscles along spine

▓ Stretches spine

▓ Builds core strength

PRECAUTIONS

▓ Spine, shoulder, arm, wrist, hip, knee, or ankle condition, injury, or pain

PROPS

▓ Yoga mat

▓ Blanket

▓ Wall

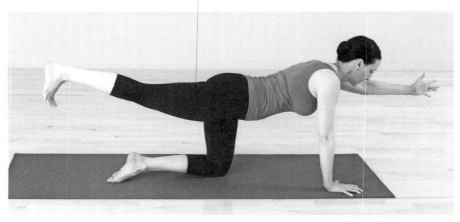

Spinal Balance Pose

POSE INSTRUCTIONS

1. Begin in Table Pose (see page 280 for instructions).

2. Extend your right leg behind your right sitting bone.

3. Pull your belly in and up, and lift your right leg to hip height.

4. Level your hips.

5. Flex your right foot and press out through your right heel, energizing the entire leg.

6. Lift and extend your left arm forward at shoulder height.

7. Point your left thumb skyward and stretch as though you are reaching for something in front of you.

8. Gaze forward and down, keeping your neck long.

9. Maintain a steady gaze about a foot in front of you, focusing on the earth.

10. Enjoy the Spinal Balance for 3 to 5 breaths.

11. Practice the instructions above using the opposite side of your body.

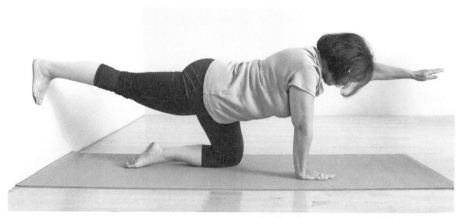

Spinal Balance Pose with foot at wall

*If you can
find spinal balance
then physical,
psychological,
and spiritual
matters are in
your control.*

LINDSAY, YOGA MOVES STUDENT

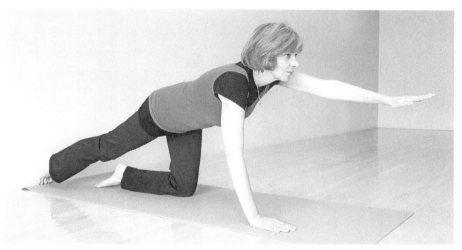

Spinal Balance Pose at the wall with back foot on earth

ADAPTATIONS AND VARIATIONS

- Place a blanket under your knees.
- Extend the right leg back with toes remaining on the earth instead of raising your leg to hip height.
- Extend the left arm forward with fingertips on the earth instead of raising your arm to shoulder height.
- Press your right foot into a wall.
- Extend only your left arm forward with both knees on the earth.
- Extend only your right leg back with both hands on the earth.

Spinal Balance Pose

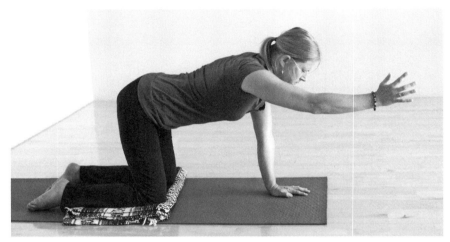

Spinal Balance Pose with arm extended forward

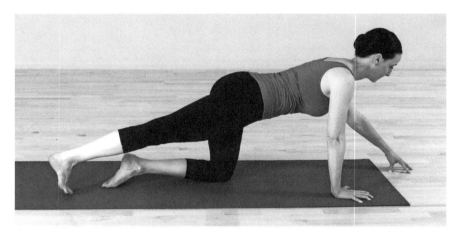

Spinal Balance Pose with fingertips, and toes touching earth

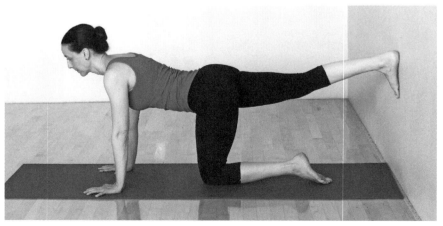

Spinal Balance Pose with hands on earth and foot pressing into wall

Spinal Twist Pose in a Chair

Bharadvajasana Variation

PRIMARY BENEFITS

■ Lengthens and lubricates spine

■ Strengthens core

■ Opens shoulders

■ Improves digestion

PRECAUTIONS

■ Spinal, shoulder, or neck condition, injury, or pain

PROPS

■ Yoga mat

■ Blanket

■ Chair

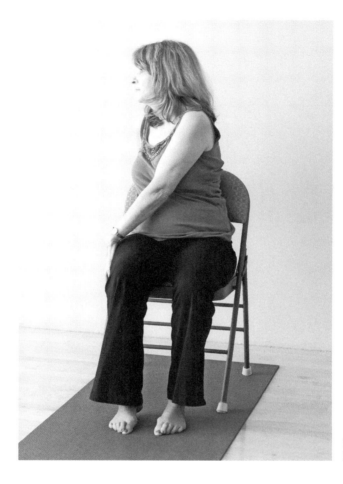

Spinal Twist
Pose in a Chair

POSE INSTRUCTIONS

1. Begin in Mountain Pose in a Chair (see page 222 for instructions).

2. Turn toward your right and place your right hand OR forearm on the back of your chair.

3. Place your left hand against the outside of your right knee. Press your knee against your hand and your hand against your knee.

4. Draw your belly in and up.

5. Begin the twist to the right from your navel and then continue the twist up your spine.

Spinal Twist Pose in a Chair

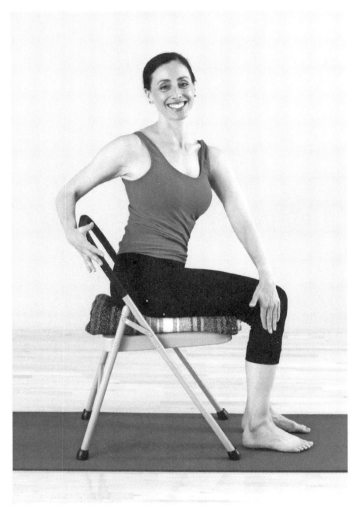

Spinal Twist
Pose in a Chair

6. Roll your right shoulder back.

7. Turn your head toward the right after you have twisted your spine. Turning your head too far to the right may strain your neck.

8. Continue to lengthen your spine and pull your belly in and up.

9. Use leverage in your hands to pull your shoulder blades together on your back. Feel your right shoulder open as you twist.

10. Enjoy Spinal Twist Pose in a Chair for 3 to 5 breaths.

11. Practice the instructions above, twisting to the opposite side of your body.

ADAPTATIONS AND VARIATIONS

- Sit on a blanket for comfort.

- Sit sideways on the right side of the chair. Place both your hands on the back of the chair. Lift through your spine and twist to the right. Extend further into the twist by pulling on the chair back while drawing your shoulder blades together down your back.

- Practice Half Lord of the Fishes Pose (see page 189 for instructions).

- Practice Sage Twist Pose (see page 255 for instructions).

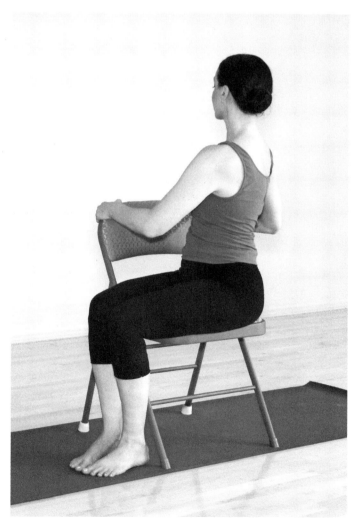

Spinal Twist Pose in a Chair seated sideways

Spinal Twist Pose Reclining

Jathara Parivartanasana

PRIMARY BENEFITS

■ Encourages spinal mobility, detoxification and hydration

■ Stimulates healthy digestion and circulation

■ Opens shoulders and heart

■ Stretches hips and spinal muscles

■ Relieves back pain and fatigue

■ Can be practiced as an active or restorative pose

PRECAUTIONS

■ Spinal condition, injury, or pain

■ Degenerative disk disease

■ Internal organ surgery

■ Pregnancy

PROPS

■ Yoga mat
■ Yoga block
■ Blanket
■ Wall

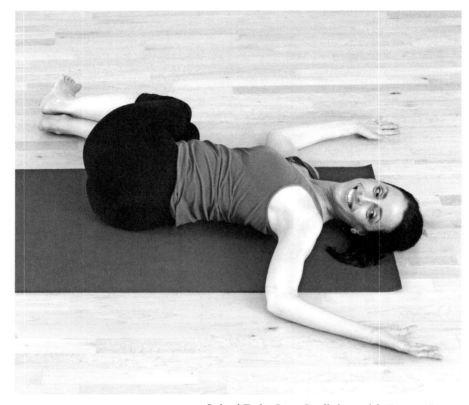

Spinal Twist Pose Reclining with "cactus" arms

POSE INSTRUCTIONS

1. Begin in Bridge Prep Pose (see page 137 for instructions).

2. Bring your knees in toward your chest and give yourself a hug with your arms around your shins.

3. Let go of your shins and place your knees over your hips with your shins parallel to the earth forming a right angle. To support your back, contract your abdominal muscles.

4. Press your knees and feet together.

5. Twist at the waist and lower your knees down toward the earth on your right side. Try to keep your shoulders toward the earth. Place your arms in a "T" OR "cactus" position.

6. Remain in the Spinal Twist Pose Reclining for 3 to 5 breaths.

7. Practice the instructions above, twisting to the opposite side of your body.

ADAPTATIONS AND VARIATIONS

- If your left elbow or shoulder lifts, place a blanket or block under it.

- If your right knee does not touch the earth, place a blanket or block underneath your right knee.

- If your left hip is tight or you have had a hip replacement, place a block between your knees.

- You may keep your neck in neutral, OR turn your head in the opposite direction of your knees, depending on the health of your cervical vertebrae.

- To deepen the twist, bring your knees closer to your right shoulder.

- To lessen the twist, lower your knees below the level of your hips.

- Practice Spinal Twist Pose Reclining against the wall with your feet pressing into the baseboard.

- Practice "Windshield Wiper" Twist Pose. Begin in Bridge Prep Pose (see page 137 for instructions), with "cactus" arms. Lower your left knee down toward center. Feel the stretch from your outer hip down your thigh. Raise left knee and lower right knee down toward center. Raise right knee and repeat sequence 3 to 5 times.

- Practice Restorative Twist over Bolster Pose (see page 249 for instructions).

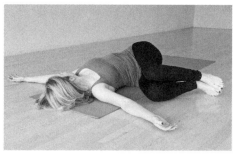

Spinal Twist Pose Reclining
with arms in "T"

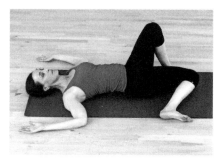

Windshield Wiper Twist Pose

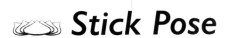 # Stick Pose

Dandasana

PRIMARY BENEFITS

■ Lengthens back of legs and spine

■ Strengthens back

■ Increases postural awareness

■ Increases inner body strength

■ Serves as foundation for other seated poses

PRECAUTIONS

■ Lower back or wrist condition, strain, injury, or pain

PROPS

■ Yoga mat

■ Yoga block

■ Yoga strap

■ Blanket

■ 2 chairs

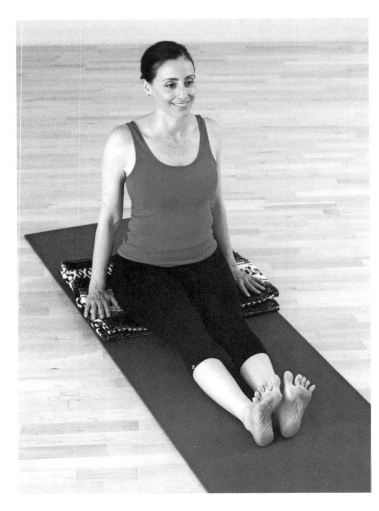

Stick Pose with blanket

POSE INSTRUCTIONS

1. Find a comfortable seated pose on the earth with your legs straight out in front of you.

2. Establish a neutral lower back curve. Lean into your left hip, place your left hand on your inner right thigh and your right hand on your outer right hip. With the left hand turn the inner thigh muscles down and with the right hand move the flesh outward and back. Repeat on your left side.

3. Place your hands on the earth at your hips for support.

4. Lift your belly in and up as you lengthen your tailbone down.

5. To lengthen the back of your legs, press your heels forward and your thighs down. Keep your knees and toes pointing upward. Notice your firm leg muscles.

6. Press down through your palms as you lengthen your torso by lifting up and out of your waist.

7. Move your shoulders over your hips, drawing the blades onto your back.

8. Draw the crown of your head skyward while keeping your eyes forward and chin level with the earth.

9. Soften your jaw and the root of your tongue.

10. Enjoy Stick Pose 3 to 5 breaths.

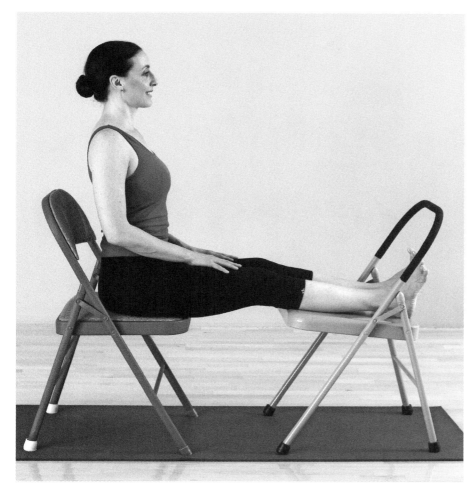

Stick Pose with two chairs, side view

Stick Pose

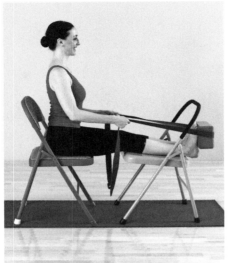
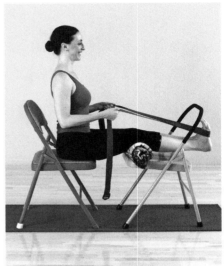

Stick Pose with two chairs, yoga strap, and block

Stick Pose with two chairs, rolled blanket, and strap

ADAPTATIONS AND VARIATIONS

- Use two chairs until you are comfortable lowering down to and rising up from the earth with ease.

- Place a blanket under your sitting bones so that your lower spine is not rounded back.

- Use a strap around the soles of your feet OR around a block placed at the soles of your feet. Hold both ends of the strap in your hands, and extend your feet into the block.

- Place a folded blanket or rolled mat under your knees to prevent them from locking.

- Add a twist while practicing the pose.

- Practice a forward fold in stick pose. Leading with your heart, hinge from the hips and begin to lean your spine forward.

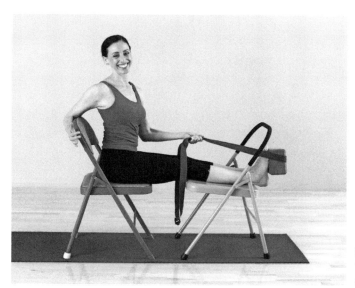

Stick Pose with twist, yoga strap, and block

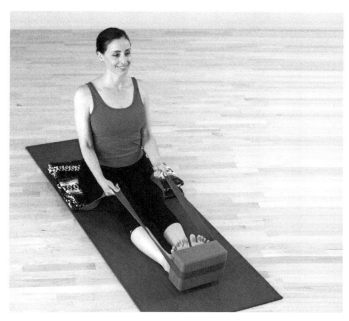

Stick Pose on blanket with strap and block

Table Pose

PRIMARY BENEFITS

■ Increases strength in upper and lower body

■ Stretches spine and torso

■ Serves as starting point for many other poses and variations

PRECAUTIONS

■ Shoulder, neck, wrist, or ankle condition, injury, or pain

PROPS

■ Yoga mat

■ Yoga dumbbells

■ Rolled mat or wedge

■ Blankets

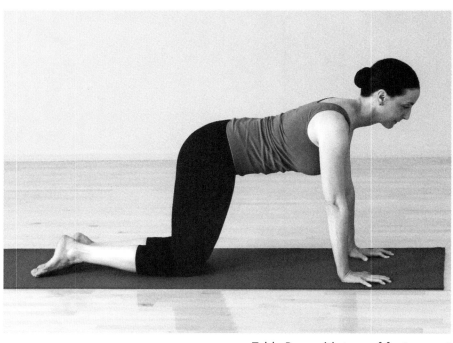

Table Pose with tops of feet on mat

POSE INSTRUCTIONS

1. Begin on the earth on your hands and knees. You may curl your toes under, OR press the tops of your feet into the mat.

2. Position your knees under your hips, OR slightly behind your hips.

3. Place your hands under your shoulders, OR slightly forward.

4. Spread your fingers as you press your hands into the earth. Resist sinking into your wrists. Make sure to root the base of your index fingers into the earth.

5. Position head, neck, and spine in a line parallel to the earth. Gaze at the earth slightly forward of fingertips.

6. Draw your shoulder blades together on your back.

7. Lengthen your tailbone toward the earth, and pull your belly in and up.

8. Enjoy Table Pose for 3 to 5 breaths.

ADAPTATIONS AND VARIATIONS

- Rotate your hands and arms away from your body OR rotate them inward. Notice the difference in how your shoulder blades move onto the back. Choose the hand position that facilitates moving your shoulder blades together on the back.

- Place a folded blanket under your knees for extra comfort.

- For weak wrists OR wrist discomfort: place a wedge or blankets under the heels of your hands; OR place your hands on yoga dumbbells; OR lower down onto your forearms with your elbows positioned under your shoulders; OR elevate your forearms on a pile of blankets.

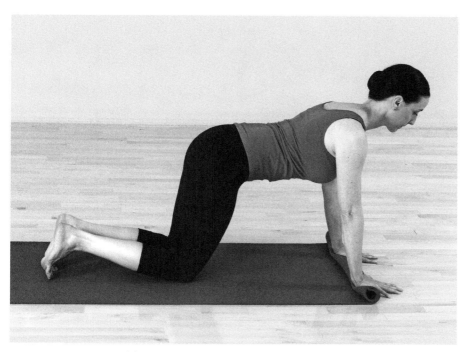

Table Pose with rolled yoga mat under hands and toes curled

Table Pose

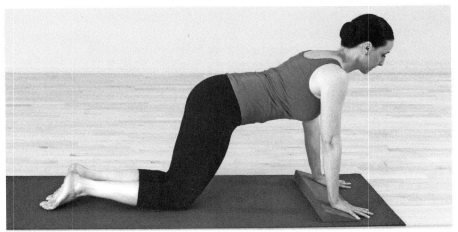

Table Pose with wedge under hands

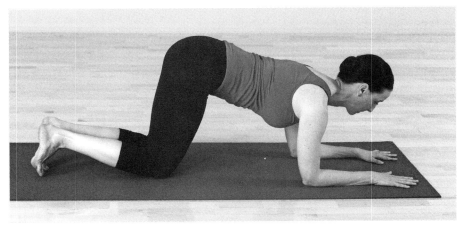

Table Pose on forearms

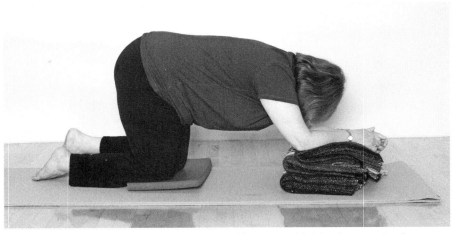

Table Pose with blankets under forearms

Table Pose with Knee to Chest

PRIMARY BENEFITS

■ Stretches legs and spine

■ Builds upper body and core strength

PRECAUTIONS

■ Shoulder, neck, wrist, or ankle condition, injury, or pain

PROPS

■ Yoga mat

■ Yoga dumbbells

■ Rolled mat or wedge

■ Blankets

■ Wall

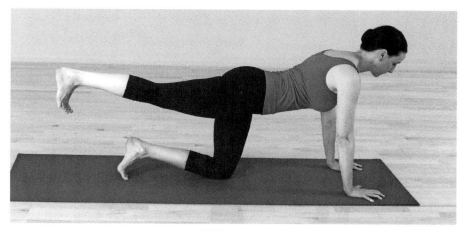

Table Pose with leg extended and flexed foot

POSE INSTRUCTIONS

1. Begin in Table Pose (see page 280 for instructions).

2. Inhale, and extend your right leg back at hip height with flexed foot.

3. Exhale, lift the belly in, and bring your right knee in toward your heart. Your spine curves upward like Cat Pose (see page 146 for photo).

4. Repeat sequence 3 to 5 times; inhaling while extending the right leg back, and exhaling while bringing the right knee in toward heart.

5. Practice the instructions above using the opposite side of your body.

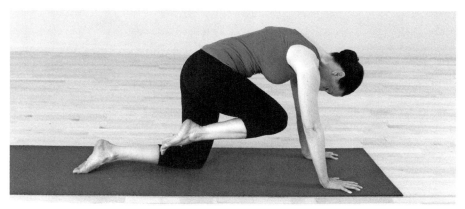

Table Pose with knee toward chest and belly lifed

Table Pose with Knee to Chest

ADAPTATIONS AND VARIATIONS

- Place a folded blanket under knees for comfort.
- Extend leg with flexed toes pressing into the earth for more support.
- Press your foot into a wall as it extends back.
- For weak wrists OR wrist discomfort: place a wedge or blankets under the heels of your hands; OR place your hands on yoga dumbbells; OR lower down onto your forearms with your elbows positioned under your shoulders; OR elevate your forearms on a pile of blankets so that your hips and shoulders are on the same plane.

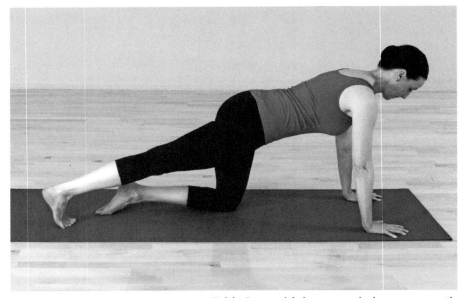

Table Pose with leg extended, toes on earth

Table Pose with Knee Circles

PRIMARY BENEFITS

■ Builds upper body strength

■ Loosens hip joints

■ Improves balance

PRECAUTIONS

■ Shoulder, neck, wrist, or ankle condition, injury, or pain

PROPS

■ Yoga mat

■ Yoga dumbbells

■ Rolled mat or wedge

■ Blankets

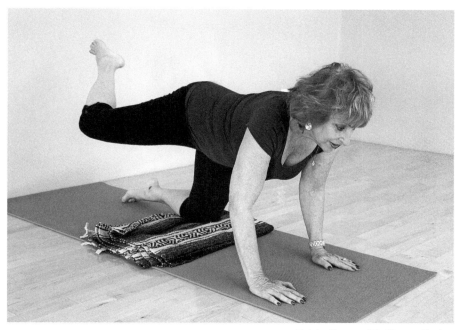

Table Pose with Knee Circles

POSE INSTRUCTIONS

1. Begin in Table Pose (see page 280 for instructions).

2. Lift your right knee.

3. Open your right knee to the right side. Make small circles with your knee, gradually increasing circle size according to your range of motion.

4. Repeat circling motion 3 to 5 times.

5. Practice the instructions above using the opposite side of your body.

ADAPTATIONS AND VARIATIONS

• Place a folded blanket under your knees for comfort.

• For weak wrists OR wrist discomfort: place a wedge or blankets under the heels of your hands; OR place your hands on yoga dumbbells; OR lower down onto your forearms with your elbows positioned under your shoulders; OR elevate your forearms on a pile of blankets so that your hips and shoulders are on the same plane.

Table Pose in Reverse

Purvottanasana Variation

PRIMARY BENEFITS

■ Lengthens front of body

■ Strengthens core, upper body, back, buttocks, legs, arms, wrists, and neck

PRECAUTIONS

■ Neck, shoulder, or wrist condition, injury, or pain

PROPS

■ Yoga mat

■ Yoga block

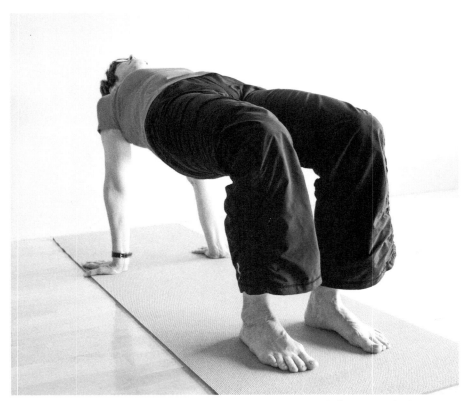

Table Pose in Reverse with fingers pointing away

POSE INSTRUCTIONS

1. Sit on the earth with your knees bent and your feet about a foot in front of your hips, aligning your knees and toes, so they are pointing straight forward.

2. Place your hands behind your hips with your fingers pointing out to the sides.

3. Press into the earth with your hands and feet.

4. Lift your hips and heart until your thighs and torso are parallel to the earth. Draw your shoulder blades together on your back.

5. Tone your buttocks, and extend your tailbone toward your knees.

6. Tuck your chin toward your chest. Gently roll your head back until your head, neck, and heart are in line.

7. Enjoy Table Pose in Reverse for 3 to 5 breaths.

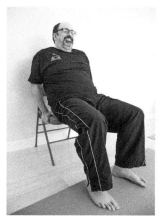

Table Pose in Reverse with
a chair and bent knees

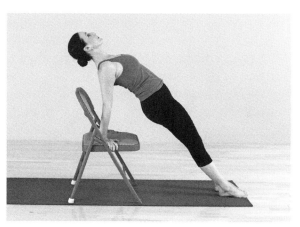

Table Pose in Reverse with chair
and with straight knees

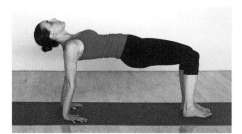

Table Pose in Reverse
with fingers toward feet

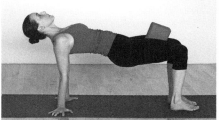

Table Pose in Reverse with block
between thighs and fingers
pointing to the sides

ADAPTATIONS AND VARIATIONS

- Practice alternate hand position with fingers pointing toward your feet, OR away from you.
- Hold for increasingly longer times to build endurance.
- Hold a yoga block between your thighs to feel your core as you lift into the pose.
- Practice with a chair with knees bent or straight.
- Practice Bridge Pose (see page 137 for instructions).

Thigh Stretch Pose on the Earth

PRIMARY BENEFITS

■ Lengthens front of thighs and hip flexors

■ Releases lower back tension

■ Opens hips

■ Opens shoulder

■ Improves balance when practicing Thigh Stretch Pose on the side variation

PRECAUTIONS

■ Neck, shoulder, or wrist condition, injury, or pain

PROPS

■ Yoga mat

■ Yoga strap

■ Blanket

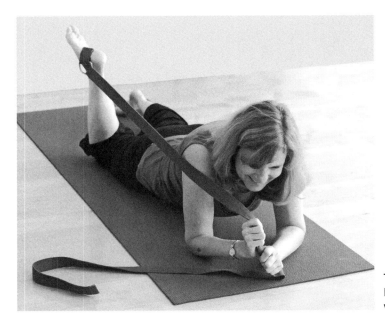

Thigh Stretch Pose on belly with strap

POSE INSTRUCTIONS

1. Make a small loop in your strap for your foot and place it by your side on the mat.

2. Begin on your belly in Sphinx Pose (see page 266 for instructions).

3. Bend your right knee with your foot facing skyward.

4. Place a looped strap around your right foot, OR clasp your right hand around your right foot.

5. Keep your knees close together so that your knees are lined up with your sitting bones.

6. Draw your foot toward your right buttocks until you feel a gentle stretch along the front of your right thigh.

7. If holding foot with your hand instead of a strap, press your right foot into your right hand, and press your hand into your foot.

8. Extend your tailbone back toward your heels while your belly lifts in and up.

9. Enjoy Thigh Stretch Pose on the Earth for 3 to 5 breaths.

10. Practice the instructions above using the opposite side of your body.

ADAPTATIONS AND VARIATIONS

- When using the yoga strap, experiment with elbow placement by placing the elbow on the earth or pointing it forward.

- If you cannot raise up on your forearms, place your forehead down on your left hand before reaching for your right foot.

- Place a blanket under your pelvis to reduce pressure on the lower back and to cushion your hips.

- If you need assistance, ask a friend to place the loop on your foot for you.

- For a shoulder opener and more intense thigh stretch, square your shoulders toward the front of the mat when holding foot or strap.

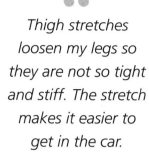

Thigh stretches loosen my legs so they are not so tight and stiff. The stretch makes it easier to get in the car.

ANNE, YOGA MOVES STUDENT

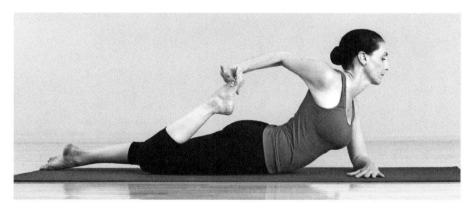

Thigh Stretch Pose on forearms with hand on foot

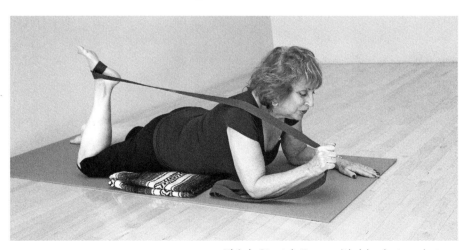

Thigh Stretch Pose with blanket and strap

Thigh Stretch Pose on the Earth

- Practice Thigh Stretch Pose on the side:
  1. Lie on your right side with your head resting on your right arm.
  2. Bend your right knee to balance your torso.
  3. Bend your left knee in front of your belly and place your left hand on your left ankle or foot.
  4. Line up your left knee with your hip.
  5. Draw your foot toward your left buttocks until you feel a gentle stretch along the front of your left thigh.
  6. Press your left foot into your left hand, and press your hand into your foot.
  7. Keep your left elbow bent to access an increased range of motion in your shoulders.

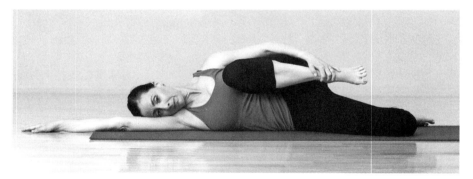

Thigh Stretch Pose on the side, preparation

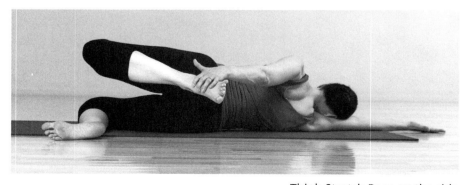

Thigh Stretch Pose on the side

Thread the Needle Pose

Parivrtta Balasana

PRIMARY BENEFITS

■ Improves flexibility of spine

■ Strengthens core

■ Opens shoulders

■ Improves balance, digestion, and mood

PRECAUTIONS

■ Spine, neck, knee, or shoulder condition, injury, or pain

PROPS

■ Yoga mat

■ Yoga block

■ Blanket

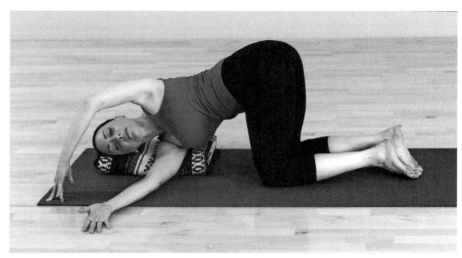

Thread the Needle Pose

POSE INSTRUCTIONS

1. Begin in Table Pose (see page 280 for instructions).
2. Stretch your right arm out to the side and raise it skyward.
3. Circle your right arm down and slide your forearm behind your left wrist.
4. Roll onto your right shoulder as you slide your right arm further to the left.
5. Press into the earth with your left fingertips.
6. Enjoy Thread the Needle Pose for 3 to 5 breaths.
7. Practice the instructions above using the opposite side of your body.

ADAPTATIONS AND VARIATIONS

- Place a folded blanket under your right shoulder.
- Extend your left leg back and press your toes into the earth.
- Extend and lift your left leg.
- Rotate your left arm toward your feet and behind your back, pressing the back of your left hand into your back.

Thread the Needle Pose

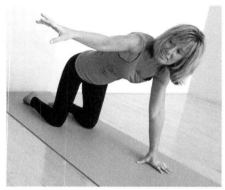

Thread the Needle Pose
preparation with arm lifted

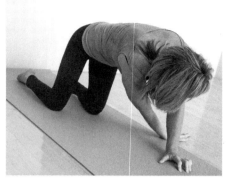

Thread the Needle Pose
preparation with arm lowered
behind opposite wrist

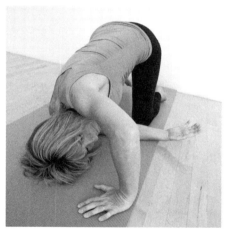

Thread the Needle Pose

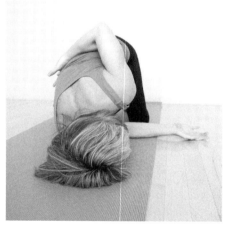

Thread the Needle Pose
with left hand behind

Tree Pose

Vrksasana

PRIMARY BENEFITS

■ Calms nervous system

■ Lengthens and strengthens legs, hips, and spinal muscles

■ Improves balance and focus

■ Opens inner thigh muscles and hips

PRECAUTIONS

■ Balance concerns

■ Foot, ankle, knee, hip condition, injury, or pain

PROPS

■ Yoga mat

■ Chair

■ Wall

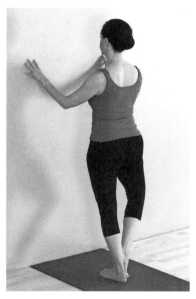
"Baby Bush" Pose

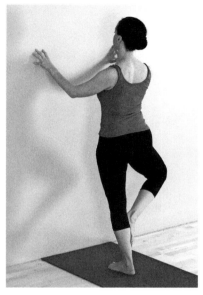
"Shrub" Pose at wall

POSE INSTRUCTIONS

1. Begin in Mountain Pose (see page 220 for instructions) facing the wall.

2. Place your fingertips on the wall for this balancing pose.

3. Shift your weight onto your left leg. Raise your right heel with your knee pointing forward.

4. Rotate your right knee to the right and place your right foot at your left ankle for "Baby Bush" Pose.

5. Level your hips.

6. Press your right foot and your left ankle into each other to find your center.

7. Press down through your left leg and tone the leg and hip muscles as you lift skyward through your spine.

8. Pull your belly in and up, and lengthen your tailbone down.

9. Find a point to focus your gaze, either on the earth, OR forward. This will help your balance.

10. Enjoy Tree Pose for 3 to 5 breaths.

11. Practice the instructions above using the opposite side of your body.

Tree Pose

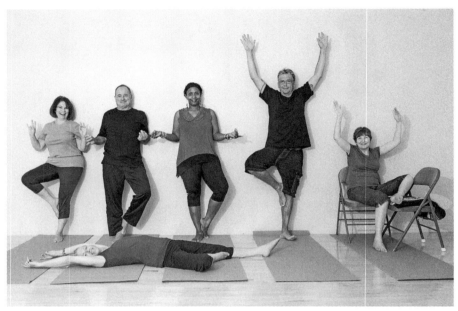

Tree Pose in the forest

ADAPTATIONS AND VARIATIONS

- Practice your balance by taking one or both hands off the wall.
- Practice Tree Pose with your back to the wall.
- Place your right foot at your left shin ("Shrub" Pose), OR at your left inner thigh for Tree Pose. Do not place your right foot at your left knee joint. You may use your right hand to help you place your right foot on your left inner thigh.
- Practice Tree Pose with your right foot on a chair beside you.
- Practice Tree Pose with your right knee pressed into wall.
- Practice Tree Pose in the middle of your mat in the following ways: next to or behind a chair with one or both hands on your hips; OR with your hands in *Anjali Mudra* or *Chin Mudra* (see pages 326 or 328 respectively for instructions); OR with your arms up overhead, palms facing one another like branches.
- Practice Tree Pose lying on the earth.
- Practice Tree Pose in a chair (see page 298 for instructions).
- Practice Tree Pose Seated on the Earth (see page 296 for instructions).

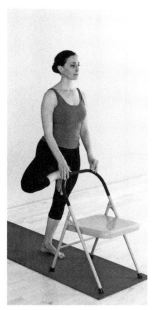
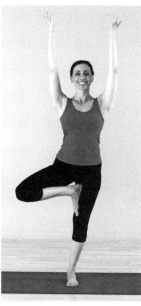
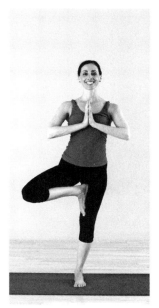

Tree Pose standing
in back of a chair

Tree Pose with arms
overhead

Tree Pose with hands
in Prayer Mudra

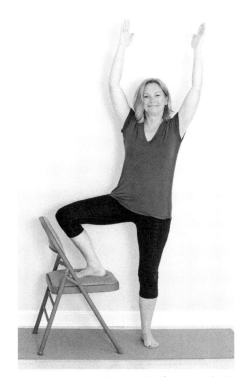
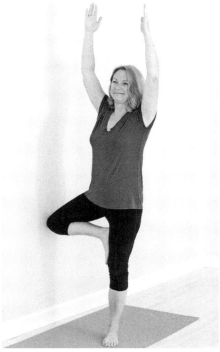

Tree Pose with foot on chair

Tree Pose with knee at wall

Tree Pose Seated on the Earth

Janu Sirsasana

PRIMARY BENEFITS

■ Calms nervous system

■ Lengthens and strengthens legs and spinal muscles

■ Stretches inner thigh muscles

■ Improves digestion

PRECAUTIONS

■ Spine, knee, hip, leg, ankle condition, injury, or pain

PROPS

■ Yoga mat

■ Yoga strap

■ Yoga block

■ 1 to 3 chairs

■ Blanket

■ Washcloth

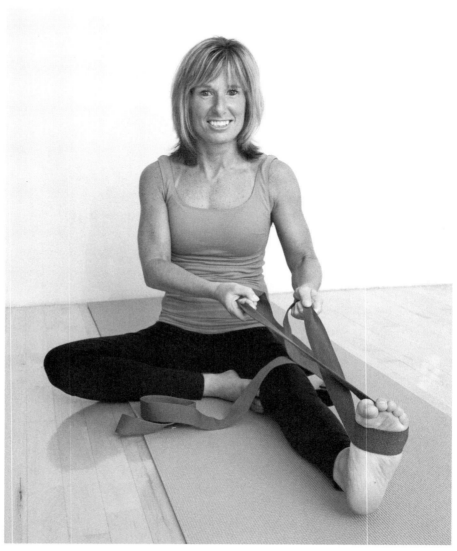

Tree Pose Seated on Earth with crossed strap

POSE INSTRUCTIONS

1. Begin in Stick Pose (see page 276 for instructions).

2. Press your left leg into the earth and flex your foot.

3. Place a strap around the arch or ball of your left foot. You may cross the strap in front of your foot for an easier grip. Notice that the placement of the strap may impact whether you feel the stretch in your hamstrings or your calf.

4. Bend the right leg with the knee pointing upward.

5. Rotate knee outward to your right side and down to the earth.

6. Press your right foot into your left inner thigh or calf, and the left thigh or calf into the sole of your right foot.

7. Lengthen skyward through your spine as you pull on the strap.

8. Bend from your hips, without rounding your spine or shoulders, until you feel a stretch through the back of your spine, legs and hips.

9. Enjoy Tree Pose Seated on the Earth for 3 to 5 breaths.

10. Practice the instructions above using the opposite side of your body.

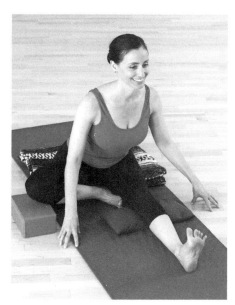

Tree Pose Seated on the Earth with blanket, block and pad

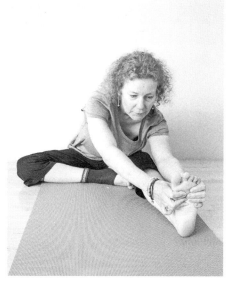

Tree Pose Seated on the Earth with hands on foot

Tree Pose Seated on the Earth

ADAPTATIONS AND VARIATIONS

- Raise your hips on a blanket.

- Support your right knee with a blanket OR block if, when lowered, your right knee is higher than your hip.

- Relieve knee discomfort with a folded washcloth placed in the "V" behind your bent right knee. If the discomfort is not relieved, exit the pose.

- Place a rolled blanket under your straight left leg if your extended knee locks.

- Practice the pose without a strap with hands on your foot, OR shin, OR on each side of your left leg.

- Place the back of a chair in front of you for support as you fold forward.

- Practice Tree Pose with three chairs. Sit in one chair and extend your left leg to a second chair in front of you. You may support the bent right knee with a third chair out to the side.

- Practice the Tree Pose in a chair:

  1. Begin in Mountain Pose in a Chair (see page 222 for instructions).

  2. Lift your right leg with a bent knee.

  3. Rotate your right knee outward, and place the right foot into the left inner thigh, OR calf, OR ankle.

  4. Press your right foot and left leg into each other.

  5. Press your left foot into the earth, as you lift your arms overhead like branches on a tree.

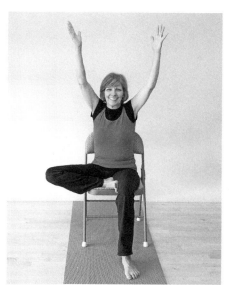

Tree Pose in chair

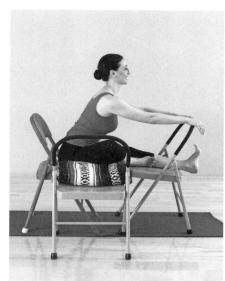

Tree Pose with three chairs and blanket

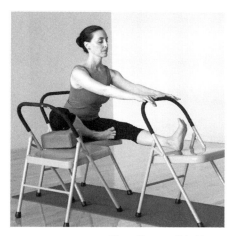

Tree Pose with three
chairs and block

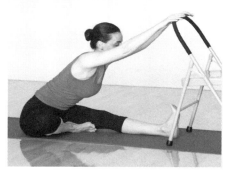

Tree Pose Seated on the
Earth with hands on chair,
and forward fold

Triangle Pose

Utthita Trikonasana

PRIMARY BENEFITS

▓ Strengthens legs
and core

▓ Stretches spine, sides
of body, shoulders,
hamstrings, inner thighs,
calves and ankles

▓ Improves breathing

▓ Lessens effects
of scoliosis

PRECAUTIONS

▓ Balance concerns

▓ Neck, hip, knee, ankle
condition, injury, or pain

PROPS

▓ Yoga mat

▓ Yoga block

▓ 1 to 2 chairs

▓ Wall

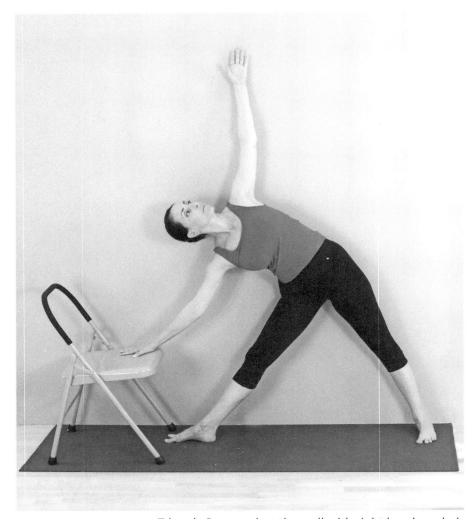

Triangle Pose against the wall with right hand on chair

POSE INSTRUCTIONS

1. Place the long side of your mat against the wall. Place a chair
on the mat with its side to the wall.

2. Begin in Mountain Pose with your back near the wall (see page
220 for instructions). The seat of the chair is to your right.

3. Place your hands on your hips.

4. Open your legs wide, 2 to 4 feet apart depending upon your
balance. Keep your legs straight but be certain not to lock
your knees.

5. Rotate your right foot 90 degrees to the right. Track your right knee over your middle toes.

6. Turn your left toes slightly in toward your center to help your balance.

7. Press down firmly through the big toe mounds of your feet.

8. Pull your feet either toward each other, OR away from each other. Side bend by hinging from your hips to the right. Reach out and place your right hand to the chair.

9. Pull your belly in and up, and lengthen down through your tailbone.

10. Lift your left arm skyward and gaze forward OR toward your left hand.

11. Keep your hips at the wall, align your head, shoulders, and hips, and lengthen your spine.

12. Feel a stretch along the left side of your body.

13. Enjoy Triangle Pose for 3 to 5 breaths.

14. Return your left hand to your left hip and press down through both feet to rise. Place your right hand on your right hip, returning to a wide-legged stance, with feet facing forward.

15. Move the chair to opposite end of mat and practice the instructions above using the opposite side of your body.

Triangle Pose

ADAPTATIONS AND VARIATIONS

- Place your right hand on your shin, OR your ankle, OR a block, OR the earth.
- Place the short end of the mat against the wall and the chair at the opposite end. Place your left heel against the wall for stability. Side bend toward the chair, and place your right hand on the seat of the chair.
- Place the short end of the mat against the wall and the chair back against the wall. Side bend toward the chair, and place your right hand on the seat of the chair.

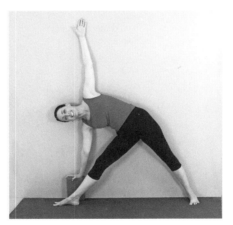

Triangle Pose against wall with right hand on block

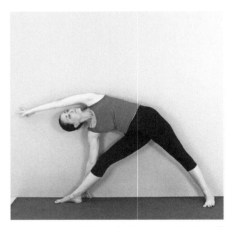

Triangle Pose against wall with arm extended over ear

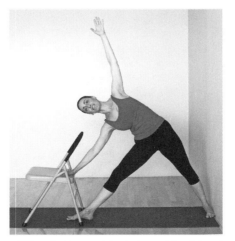

Triangle Pose with chair and back heel pressing into wall

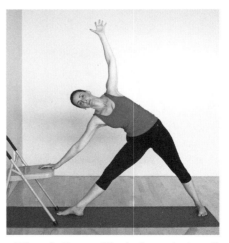

Triangle Pose with chair against wall and right hand on chair

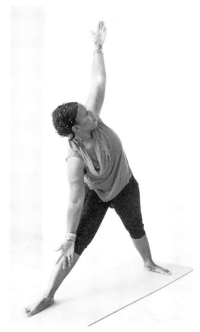

Triangle Pose
in the middle
of mat

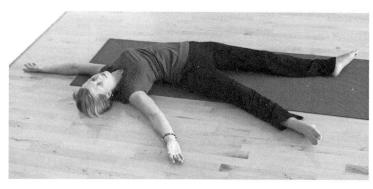

Triangle Pose
on the earth

- Practice Triangle Pose in the middle of your mat.
- Practice Triangle Pose on the earth:
  1. Begin in Mountain Pose on the Earth (see page 221 for instructions).
  2. Widen the right leg out to the side.
  3. Place your arms in a "T."
  4. Side bend to the right at your hips.
  5. Reach your right arm in the direction of your right foot.
  6. Feel a stretch along the left side of your body.

Triangle Pose

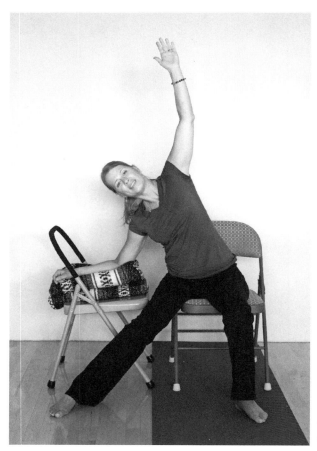

Triangle Pose
with two chairs

- Practice Triangle Pose with two chairs:
  1. Place one chair on the mat and another chair to the right with folded blankets on the seat.
  2. Sit in the chair on the mat and sit toward the front of the seat.
  3. Lengthen your right leg out to your side in front of the right chair.
  4. Side bend to the right and place your right forearm on the folded blankets.
  5. Lift your left arm skyward and feel a stretch along the left side of your body.
  6. Enjoy Triangle Pose with two Chairs for 3 to 5 breaths.
- Practice Side Plank Pose, Variation 3: Gate Pose (see page 263)

Wall Dog Pose

Adho Mukha Svanasana Variation

PRIMARY BENEFITS

▧ Strengthens and lengthens spine, legs, and arms

▧ Open shoulders

PRECAUTIONS

▧ Balance concerns

▧ Spine, shoulder, wrist, knee condition, injury, or pain

PROPS

▧ Yoga mat

▧ Yoga block

▧ Yoga dumbbells

▧ Chair

▧ Wall

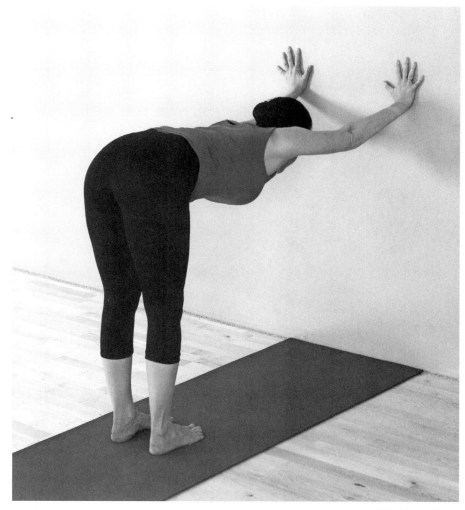

Wall Dog Pose

POSE INSTRUCTIONS

1. Stand in Mountain Pose (see page 220 for instructions) facing a wall.

2. Firmly press your hands into the wall at shoulder height and shoulder distance.

3. Walk your feet back until you form an "L" and feel a stretch in your arms, shoulders, spine, or legs.

4. Adjust your hands so that your arms are in line with your ears.

5. Enjoy Wall Dog Pose for 3 to 5 breaths.

Wall Dog Pose

ADAPTATIONS AND VARIATIONS

- Place a block between your thighs, contract them to feel your strong core.

- Practice using yoga dumbbells to assist weak wrists.

- If your hamstrings and lower back are tight, bend your knees and angle your hips high to find the lower back curve as in Cow Pose (see page 146 for photo). Remain here or begin to straighten your legs while maintaining the lower back curve.

- Practice Wall Dog Pose standing with a chair. Place a chair back against the wall. Begin standing and place your hands on the chair seat. Walk your feet back until you form an "L" with your body.

- Practice Wall Dog Pose on knees with a chair. Place a chair back against the wall. Begin on your hands and knees. Place your hands on the chair with your arms outstretched.

- Practice Wall Dog Pose sitting in a chair. Sit in a chair facing a wall. Place your arms above your head in line with your ears and press your hands into the wall.

- Practice Downward Facing Dog Pose (see page 170 for instructions).

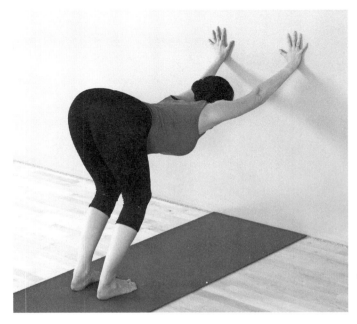

Wall Dog Pose with
bent knees and
lower back curve

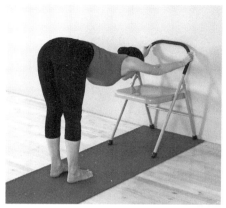

Wall Dog Pose with
chair at wall

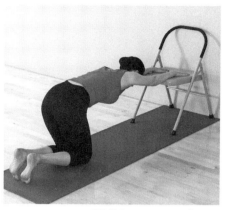

Wall Dog Pose on knees
with chair at wall

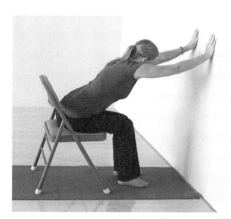

Wall Dog Pose in chair

Warrior 2 Pose

Virabhadrasana II

PRIMARY BENEFITS

■ Strengthens legs, arms, inner thighs, and core

■ Opens hips, shoulders, hamstrings, and inner thighs

■ Improves balance

■ Builds focus, confidence, and energy

PRECAUTIONS

■ Balance concerns

■ Ankle, knee, inner thigh, groin, or hip condition, injury, or pain

PROPS

■ Yoga mat

■ Yoga block

■ Chair

■ Wall

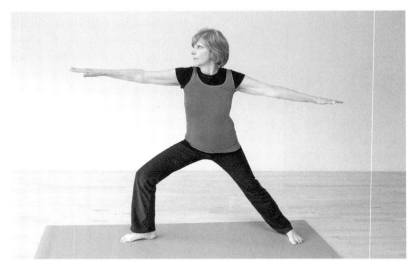

Warrior 2 Pose

POSE INSTRUCTIONS

1. Begin in Mountain Pose (see page 220 for instructions) facing the long side of the mat.

2. Place your hands on your hips, and step your feet 2 to 4 feet apart, with your legs wide. Be careful not to lock your knees.

3. Turn your right foot out 90 degrees, toward the top of the mat, and turn your left foot slightly in for balance.

4. Bend your right knee over your middle toes, and keep your left leg straight.

5. Press down through both feet, and lengthen through your spine.

6. Lift your arms into a "T," and press your shoulder blades together on your back, as you lengthen out through your arms and fingers.

7. Gaze toward your right hand while keeping your torso facing the long side of the mat.

8. Enjoy the Warrior 2 Pose for 3 to 5 breaths.

9. Return to a wide-legged stance with toes facing the long side of your mat.

10. Practice the instructions above using the opposite side of your body.

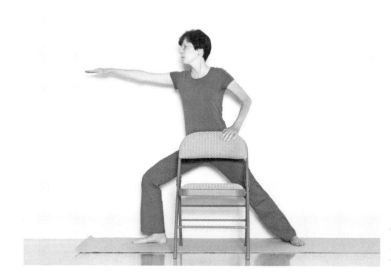

Warrior 2 Pose
against wall
with chair

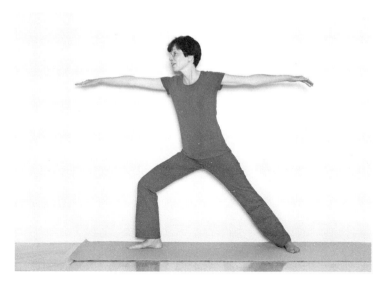

Warrior 2 Pose
against wall

Warrior 2 Pose

ADAPTATIONS AND VARIATIONS

- Practice Warrior 2 Pose with your back against the wall.

- Practice Warrior 2 Pose with your back against a wall and one or both of your hands on a chair in front of you.

- Hug your feet toward each other, OR press them away from each other, OR alternate between hugging in and pressing out your feet to build strength and stability.

- Practice Warrior 2 Pose with your right knee pointed to the wall, and place a block between the wall and your bent right knee.

- Practice Reverse Warrior 2 Pose. Press your left hand into the back of your left leg and raise your right arm to the sky. Refer to photo of Reverse Warrior 2 Pose in a Chair on page 312.

- Practice a dynamic flowing movement between Warrior 2 Pose and Reverse Warrior 2 Pose up to 3 times.

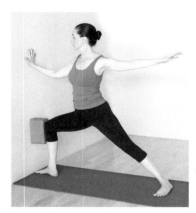

Warrior 2 Pose with block between wall and knee

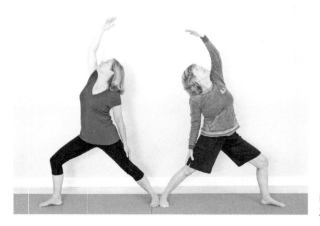

Reverse Warrior 2 Pose

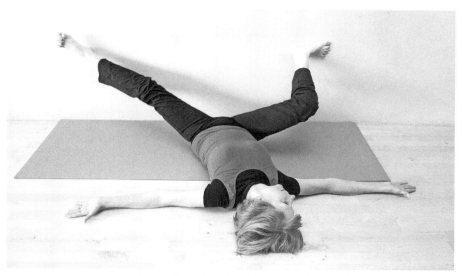

Variation: Warrior 2 Pose on the earth with feet on wall

- Practice Warrior 2 Pose on the earth:

  1. Place the long edge of the mat against the wall.

  2. Position yourself on your back with your legs on the wall (see Legs Up the Wall Pose page 212 for positioning).

  3. Bend your right knee and rotate knee to the right side. Press your foot into the wall with your knee tracking over your middle toe.

  4. Open a straight left leg out to the left side. Press your heel into the wall and flex your left foot.

  5. Open your arms into a "T" and gaze at your right hand.

Warrior 2 Pose in a Chair

Virabhadrasana II Variation

PRIMARY BENEFITS

■ Opens hips, shoulders, hamstrings, inner thighs, and core

■ Strengthens legs, arms, and inner thighs

■ Improves balance

■ Builds focus, confidence, and energy

PRECAUTIONS

■ Ankle, knee, inner thigh, groin, or hip condition, injury, or pain

PROPS

■ Yoga mat

■ Chair

■ Blankets

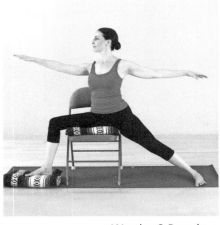

Warrior 2 Pose in a
Chair with blankets

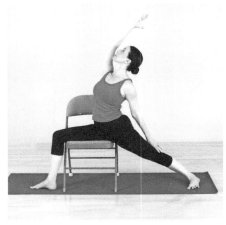

Reverse Warrior 2
Pose in a chair

POSE INSTRUCTIONS

1. Begin in Mountain Pose in a Chair (see page 222 for instructions).

2. Sit on the edge of your chair.

3. Open your right knee to your right side, and place your right heel under your knee. Track your right knee over your middle toes.

4. Straighten your left leg out to the left side with your toes on the earth and facing forward.

5. Press down firmly through both feet, and rise through your spine.

6. Spread your arms in a "T," soften your shoulders, and roll your blades onto your back.

7. Pull your belly in and up and your tailbone down.

8. Pull your feet either toward each other, OR away from each other.

9. Enjoy Warrior 2 Pose in a Chair for 3 to 5 breaths.

10. Practice the instructions above using opposite side of your body.

ADAPTATIONS AND VARIATIONS

- Place a folded blanket under your hips.

- Place a folded blanket under your right foot.

- Practice with palms facing skyward.

- Begin by placing your right sitting bone and thigh on the chair and move your left sitting bone off the chair.

- To keep right knee centered over toes, keep left arm out to the side, but press the back of your right hand into your right inner thigh.

- Hug your feet toward each other, OR press them away from each other, OR alternate between hugging in and pressing out your feet to build strength and stability.

- Practice Reverse Warrior 2 Pose in a chair. Press your left hand into your left leg and lift your right arm to the sky.

- Practice a flowing dynamic movement between Warrior 2 Pose and Reverse Warrior 2 Pose up to 3 times.

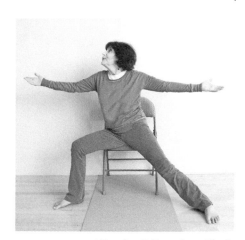

Warrior 2 Pose in a Chair

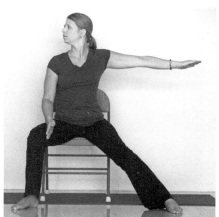

Warrior 2 Pose in a Chair with right hand pressing into right inner thigh

Warrior 3 Pose

Virabhadrasana III

PRIMARY BENEFITS

■ Improves balance

■ Strengthens back, legs, and ankles

PRECAUTIONS

■ Balance concerns

■ Leg, knee, or ankle injury, or pain

PROPS

■ Yoga mat

■ Chair

■ Wall

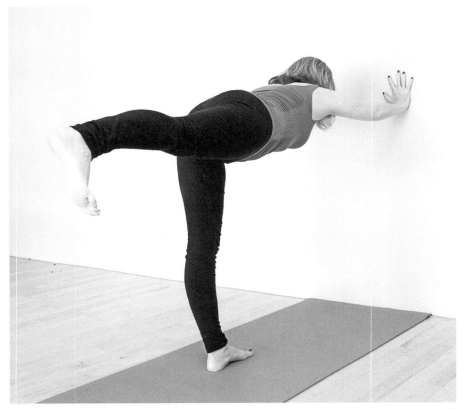

Warrior 3 Pose with hands on wall

POSE INSTRUCTIONS

1. Begin in Wall Dog Pose (see page 305 for instructions).

2. Extend your right leg behind you. Pull your belly in and up and raise your right leg to hip height. Flex your right foot.

3. Level your hips by rotating the outside of your right hip toward the earth.

4. Press strongly into the earth through your left leg and through the left toe mound. Be careful not to lock your left knee.

5. Lengthen your tailbone toward your heels and continue to draw your belly in and up.

6. Enjoy Warrior 3 Pose for 3 to 5 breaths.

7. Lower your right leg and return to Wall Dog Pose.

8. Practice the instructions above using the opposite side of your body.

ADAPTATIONS AND VARIATIONS

- Practice Warrior 3 Pose at a wall with the front of a chair against the wall. Place your hands on the back of the chair for support.

- Practice your balance in Warrior 3 Pose by releasing your fingertips from the wall or chair in front of you, OR extending your arms to the side in a "T" like an airplane.

- Practice variations of Spinal Balance (see page 268 for instructions).

- Practice Warrior 3 Pose in the middle of your mat beginning in Crescent Warrior Pose (see page 166 for instructions).

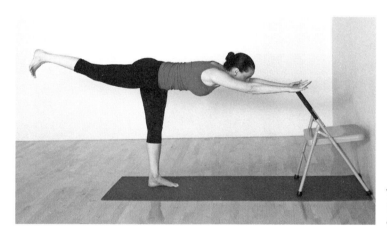

Warrior 3 Pose with chair at wall

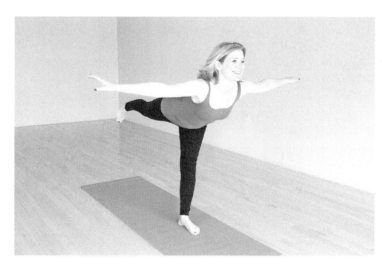

Warrior 3 Pose with arms in "T"

Wide Angle Forward Fold Pose

Upavistha Konasana

PRIMARY BENEFITS

■ Stretches spine, back of legs, and inner thighs

■ Improves sense of being grounded

PRECAUTIONS

■ Spine, hip, leg condition, injury, or pain

■ Balance concerns for standing variation

PROPS

■ Yoga mat

■ 1 to 3 chairs

■ Blankets

■ Rolled mat or washcloths

■ Wall

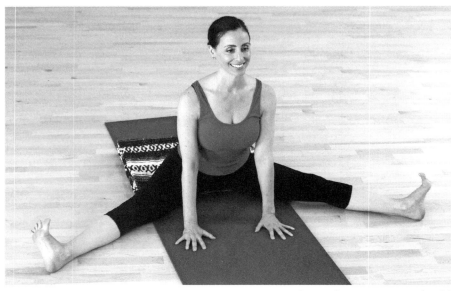

Wide Angle Pose Forward Fold

POSE INSTRUCTIONS

1. Begin in Stick Pose (see page 276 for instructions).

2. Widen your legs into a "V".

3. Establish a neutral lower back curve. Lean into your left hip, place your left hand on your inner right thigh and your right hand on your outer right hip. With the left hand turn the inner thigh muscles down and with the right hand move the flesh outward and back. Repeat on your left side.

4. Shift your weight toward the front of the sitting bones. Press your thighs toward the earth with your palms, lift up and out of your waist and hips, and lengthen your spine.

5. Draw your belly in and up, and your tailbone down.

6. Flex, point, or "floint" your feet.

7. Place your hands on the earth in front of your thighs. Lean forward until you feel a leg or back stretch. Resist the temptation to round your back to bring the head closer to the earth. Maintain the alignment of the spine from your tailbone to your crown.

8. Enjoy Wide Angle Forward Fold Pose for 3 to 5 breaths or more.

ADAPTATIONS

- Place a blanket under your hips to ensure a forward pelvic tilt and comfort.

- If your knees lock or hyperextend place a rolled mat, blanket, OR washcloth under each knee.

- Alternate 5 repetitions of first simultaneously bending your knees while flexing your feet, and then simultaneously straightening your knees while pointing your toes.

- Practice Wide Angle Forward Fold Pose with a side bend. Anchor your left hip down, and raise your left arm over your left ear and bend to your right.

- Practice Restorative Wide Angle Forward Fold Pose. Rest your head on folded arms over the seat of a chair, OR a bolster and folded blanket.

- Practice Wide Angle Forward Fold Pose reclining. Begin in Legs Up the Wall Pose (see page 212 for instructions). Open legs into a "V".

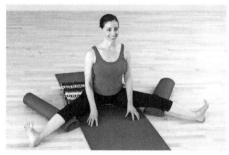

Wide Angle Forward Fold Pose with rolled mats and blanket

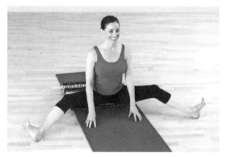

Wide Angle Forward Fold Pose with bent knees and flexed feet

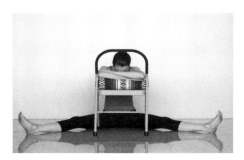

Restorative Wide Angle Forward Fold Pose over a chair seat and blanket

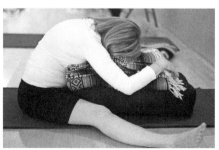

Restorative Wide Angle Forward Fold Pose over bolster and blankets

'Can you take your legs wide, like a big V?' she says. The spasticity in my legs resists, but eventually they spread and stay put. I am hit by a rush of something, something feels strange, something….'Matt, can you put your hands on your thighs, lift your chest, and breathe?' The rush intensifies. I feel something, like I am floating – no flying. Suddenly, it hits me. This is the first time in over twelve years that my legs have been wide."

MATTHEW SANFORD,
WAKING: A MEMOIR OF TRAUMA AND TRANSCENDENCE

Wide Angle Forward Fold Pose

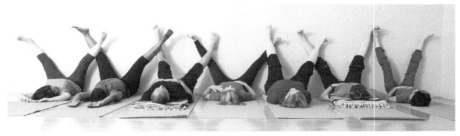

Wide Angle Forward Fold Pose reclining with legs in a "V" on wall

VARIATION 1: WIDE ANGLE FORWARD FOLD WITH THREE CHAIRS

1. Place three chairs in a triangle facing each other, and approximately 1 to 2 feet away from each other.

2. Sit in one chair.

3. Place each of your legs on the chairs that are on a diagonal to you on your left and right sides.

4. Press your palms into a block and lift it skyward with straight arms. You may also lean forward in this pose with belly engaged, OR lean into a side bend.

5. Enjoy the Wide Angle Forward Fold for 3 to 5 breaths.

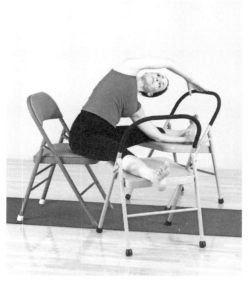

Variation 1: Wide Angle Forward Fold with Three Chairs and side bend

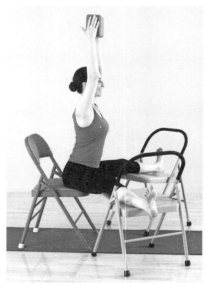

Variation 1: Wide Angle Forward Fold with Three Chairs and arms overhead

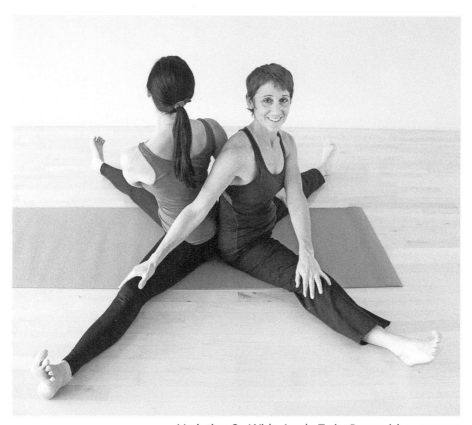

Variation 2: Wide Angle Twist Pose with a partner

VARIATION 2: WIDE ANGLE TWIST POSE
WITH A PARTNER

1. Sit back to back with a partner in Wide Angle Pose.

2. Lift through your spine and place your right hand on your partner's left thigh.

3. Place the palm of your left hand against the outside of your right thigh.

4. Press your thigh against your hand and your hand against your thigh, and twist from the navel, to your right.

5. Roll your right shoulder open.

6. Allow your head to follow turning only as far as is comfortable.

7. Enjoy the twist for 3 to 5 breaths on each side.

Wide Angle Forward Fold Pose

VARIATION 3: WIDE ANGLE FORWARD FOLD POSE WITH A PARTNER

1. Sit back to back with your partner in Wide Angle Pose.

2. Interlace elbows with your partner.

3. Take turns leaning forward and backward.

4. Enjoy each fold for 3 to 5 breaths.

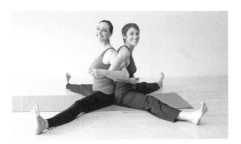
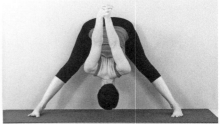

Variation 3: Wide Angle Forward Fold Pose with a partner

Variation 4: Wide Angle Forward Fold Pose Standing with interlaced fingers

VARIATION 4: WIDE ANGLE FORWARD FOLD POSE STANDING

Prasarita Padottanasana

1. Place the long edge of a mat against the wall.

2. Stand in the center of your mat with your back to the wall.

3. Spread your legs 2 to 4 feet apart depending on your balance and flexibility. Face your toes forward with your feet parallel to the short edges of your mat.

4. With your hands on your hips, begin to hinge at the hips to fold forward.

5. Hug your feet toward each other, OR press them away from each other, OR alternate between hugging in and pressing out your feet to build strength and stability.

6. You may place your hands on the earth. OR, interlace your fingers behind your back, roll your shoulder blades together on your back, and straighten your arms away from you and skyward.

7. Enjoy the pose for 3 to 5 breaths.

Yoga Squat Pose

Malasana

PRIMARY BENEFITS

- Lengthens spine and backs of legs

- Stretches pelvic floor, groin areas, thighs, and ankles

PRECAUTIONS

- Balance concerns

- Lower back, hip, knee, or ankle condition, injury, or pain

PROPS

- Yoga mat
- 1 to 2 chairs
- Blanket
- Wall

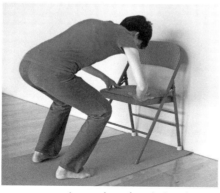

Lowering the sitting bones

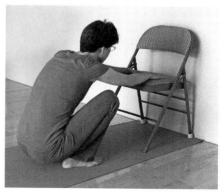

Completed Yoga Squat Pose

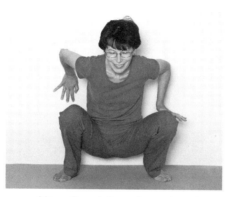

Yoga Squat Pose, lowering down while using wall for support

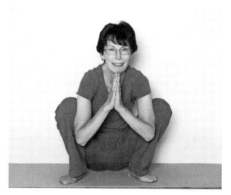

Yoga Squat Pose against wall

POSE INSTRUCTIONS

1. Place a chair and the short side of your mat against the wall.

2. Begin in Mountain Pose (see page 220 for instructions) facing the chair.

3. Place your hands on the seat of the chair.

4. Widen your stance and adjust the width depending on your flexibility, balance, and comfort. Rotate your feet and legs outward. Try a wider stance if you are new to the pose.

5. Bend your knees mindfully and deeply, keeping your knees tracking over your middle toes as you lower. You may lower your sitting bones partially, OR close to the earth. Only do what is safe and comfortable for you.

6. Enjoy Yoga Squat Pose for 3 to 5 breaths.

7. Press down on the chair to rise.

Yoga Squat Pose

ADAPTATIONS AND VARIATIONS

- Practice using a chair in front of you for support.

- Practice sitting on a block.

- Place a rolled blanket or towel under your heels if your heels rise when squatting.

- Practice Yoga Squat Pose with your back to the wall.

  1. From a wide stance, and using your hands on the wall for support, glide your hips down the wall as you bend your knees and lower your sitting bones toward the earth.

  2. Place your elbows and upper arms between your inner thighs.

  3. Hug your thighs into your arms as your elbows press back against your inner thighs.

  4. Exit Yoga Squat Pose by walking your hands forward into Table Pose, OR, exit pose by standing. Press your fingers into the mat as you lift your hips against the wall, arriving into a forward fold. When legs are straightened, lift your hands to your hips. Press down through your feet and lift your spine and head.

- Practice Yoga Squat Pose in the middle of your mat.

- Practice Goddess Pose in a Chair, OR standing variation (see page 187 for instructions).

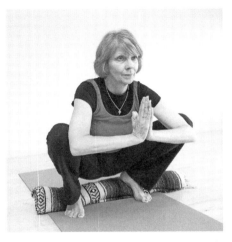

Yoga Squat with blanket under heels

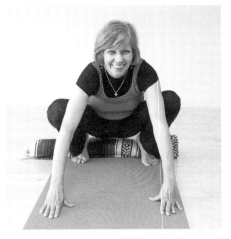

Yoga Squat with hands forward and blanket under heels

"Mudras have given me new freedom, energy, and vitality. Whether balancing in Tree Pose, or feeling the energy flow through my body when I practice the MS mudra, I experience a positive outcome. From head to toe, there are so many benefits experienced through the simple practice of placing my fingers in a mudra."

DEBORAH, YOGA MOVES STUDENT

Hand Gestures

Mudras

A *mudra* is a gesture formed by the hands or body and can represent or stimulate certain energetic qualities. It comes from the Sanskrit word *"mud"* which means "to bring joy." You may be familiar with acupuncture, acupressure or reflexology as healing methods. *Mudras* access your body's energy paths by a similar principle. When you make certain gestures, you can impact the connection between your mind, body, and spirit. The form of each *mudra* is intended to stimulate particular areas that may lead to specific sensations, emotions and physiological benefits. This "Hand Gestures" chapter offers a small sampling to introduce you to the practice.

My students fully enjoy using *mudras*,

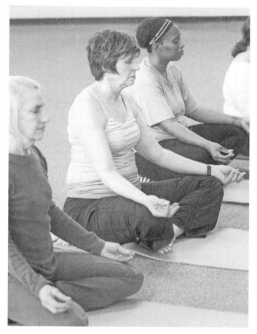

and find them accessible and empowering. You can practice *mudras* with breathing exercises (*pranayama*), with meditation, and when repeating a favorite prayer, poem, or positive affirmation. An affirmation can help you bring into your life a desired concept. For example, while holding a *mudra* repeat in your mind "I am…," then complete the affirmation with a positive statement such as, peaceful, loving, strong, fearless, balanced, in harmony, or grateful.

You hold in your hands the ability to effect change throughout your body. Stimulate your own healing energy with these *mudras*. Please see the resource section for additional information.

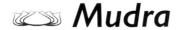 *Mudra*

PRIMARY BENEFITS

■ Stimulates energetic qualities

■ Increases mind-body connections

PRECAUTIONS

■ Dizziness

■ High blood pressure

PROPS FOR YOUR COMFORT

■ Yoga Mat

■ Chair

■ Blankets

■ Blocks

■ Anything to ensure a comfortable seat

GENERAL *MUDRA* INSTRUCTIONS

1. Choose a *mudra*.

2. Find a comfortable, centered, and well-aligned seated position such as Easy Pose, or Mountain Pose in a Chair (see pages 175 or 222, respectively, for instructions).

3. Begin with several Complete Yoga Breaths, exhaling deeply.

4. Form the hand *mudra* of your choice with a light touch of your fingers.

5. Maintain the *mudra* for 5 to 10 breaths to start. If you desire a calming effect, practice with a slow, soft breath. If you desire an energizing effect, practice with a deeper and stronger breath.

6. Gradually, as you become familiar with the *mudra*, increase your time with the *mudra*. However, some *mudra* instructions advise limiting the length of the hold. Please honor those suggestions.

7. Release the *mudra* and sit quietly. Observe your feelings or sensations.

MUDRA ADAPTATIONS AND VARIATIONS

- *Mudras* can be practiced almost anywhere and at anytime, while standing, sitting, lying in a restorative position, walking, and during a challenging conversation or situation.

- Enjoy a *mudra* at the beginning OR completion of a yoga sequence to set an intention OR seal your practice.

- Practice an affirmation, meditation, OR visualization together with a *mudra*.

- Allow the *mudra* to guide your breath pattern, OR lengthen the pauses between inhales and exhales to intensify the effect of a *mudra*.

- Many practitioners well-versed in *mudras* do not agree on an exact time to hold a *mudra* or how often to practice them. The time could vary from 5 to 10 breaths to 5 minutes. The cycle may be repeated up to 3 times per day. Often *mudra* practitioners notice that their hands and fingers are more sensitive to *mudras* the more they are practiced. Therefore, less practice time is needed to feel their effect.

- Often if you are new to a *mudra* you may feel sensation in the hands such as tingling or temperature changes. You may also enjoy a sense of well-being or calmness throughout the body. *Mudra* practitioners believe these are both positive signs. There may be an alternative *mudra* with a similar effect if you experience too much intensity or discomfort. Trust your intuition. If you are uncomfortable with a certain *mudra*, discontinue it.

Anjali (Prayer) Mudra

PRIMARY BENEFITS

■ Balances right and left hemispheres of brain, producing centering effect

SIGNIFICANCE

■ Symbolizes unity of the individual and the universal

■ Used as greeting, and to show respect, gratitude, and reverence across cultures

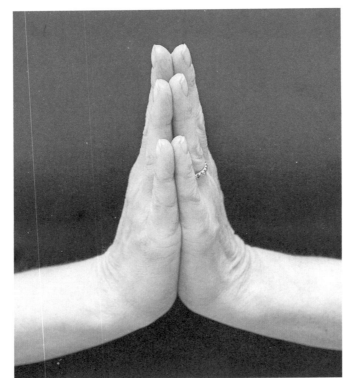

Anjali Mudra

MUDRA INSTRUCTIONS

1. Place the palms together either in front of the heart or the third eye.

2. The thumbs may touch the heart center OR the third eye, while the fingers point outward and may be together OR spread apart.

3. Enjoy *Anjali Mudra* for a few breaths OR while stating a greeting, your intention, poem, or prayer.

Bhu Mudra

PRIMARY BENEFITS

■ Reduces anxiety

■ Grounds or centers energy toward earth

■ Promotes feeling of safety

SIGNIFICANCE

■ *Bhu* means "earth"

■ Represents stability and strength of a mountain

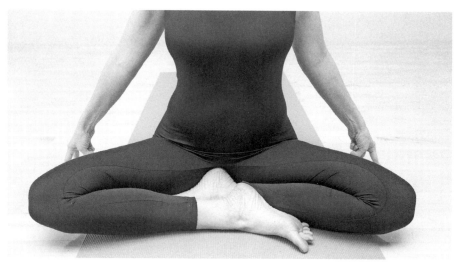

Bhu Mudra front view

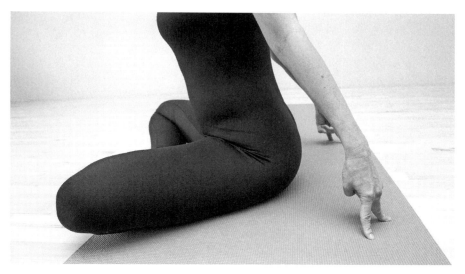

Bhu Mudra side view

MUDRA INSTRUCTIONS

1. Make the "peace" sign with both hands.

2. Place your index and middle fingers on the earth beside your hips. If you are seated in a chair, point your fingers toward the earth.

3. Enjoy *Bhu Mudra* for several breaths.

Chin Mudra

PRIMARY BENEFITS

■ Encourages concentration

■ Frequently used while meditating

SIGNIFICANCE

■ Symbolizes connection of individual and universal

■ *Chin* represents consciousness and wisdom

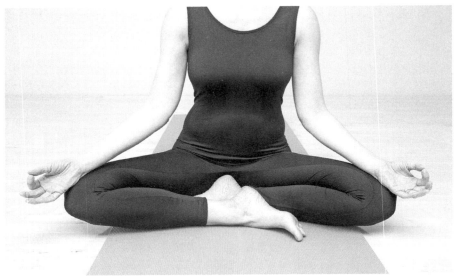

Chin Mudra facing skyward

MUDRA INSTRUCTIONS

1. Join the thumb and index finger on each hand and rest your hands on knees OR thighs.

2. The palms may face toward the earth for a calming and grounding effect, OR skyward for a receptive and open effect. *Chin Mudra* is sometimes known as *Jhana Mudra* when the palms face skyward.

3. Enjoy *Chin Mudra* for as long as desired.

Dhyana (Meditation) Mudra

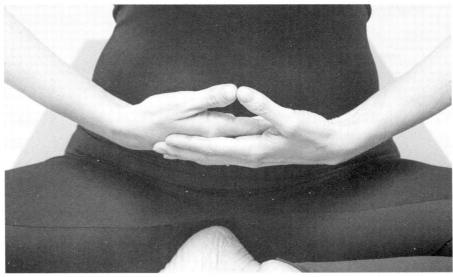

Dhyana Mudra

PRIMARY BENEFITS

■ Calms nervous system

■ Frequently used while meditating

SIGNIFICANCE

■ Represents an empty bowl waiting to be filled

MUDRA INSTRUCTIONS

1. Place your palms in front of your belly and turn palms skyward.

2. Nest the right fingers on top of the left fingers, and rest your hands in your lap.

3. Join the thumb tips together above your overlapping palms.

4. Enjoy *Dhyana Mudra* while you meditate or sit quietly.

5. You may also try the *mudra* with your left palm resting in your right palm. Perhaps you will have a different sensation.

Ganesha Mudra

PRIMARY BENEFITS

■ Invigorates heart

■ Releases tension

■ Lifts spirits

■ Builds courage to overcome obstacles

SIGNIFICANCE

■ Represents Hindu elephant diety that helps overcome obstacles

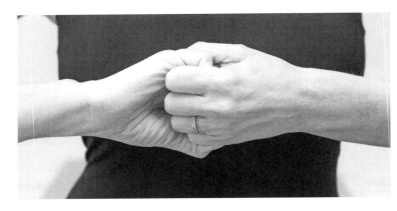

Ganesha Mudra with left hand in front of right hand

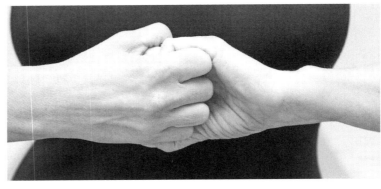

Ganesha Mudra with right hand in front of left hand

MUDRA INSTRUCTIONS

1. Place your left hand sideways in front of your heart with your fingers curled and palm facing away from you.

2. Place the right hand, with palm facing toward you, in front of the left hand. Hook your fingers together.

3. With your elbows bent to the side, inhale deeply and pull your fingers away from each other while maintaining the grip.

4. Exhale and relax your arms. Let go of any tension in your hands, arms or shoulders, without unhooking the fingers.

5. Enjoy *Ganesha Mudra*, repeating 3 to 5 times with your breath. Inhale while pulling on hooked fingers, exhale while relaxing them.

6. Repeat instructions above with hand positions reversed. Your left palm faces your heart and your right palm faces away from you.

Hakini Mudra

PRIMARY BENEFITS

■ Balances right and left hemispheres of brain

■ Improves concentration and memory

SIGNIFICANCE

■ Represents the third eye and inner wisdom

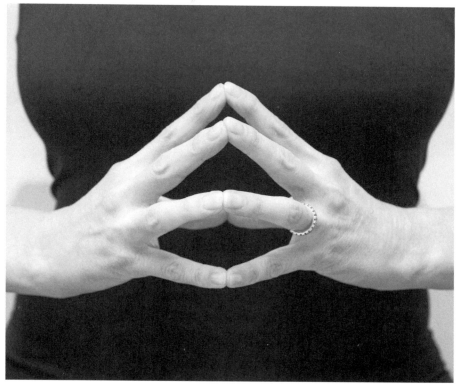

Hakini Mudra

MUDRA INSTRUCTIONS

1. Begin with your palms facing each other in front of your belly.

2. Join the fingertips of your right hand and your left hand. The palms are about four inches apart and cupped. Imagine a ball in the space between your hands.

3. Place your hands in the *mudra* in front of your belly.

4. Enjoy *Hakini Mudra* for several breaths throughout the day when you need to focus your thoughts.

Heart Centering Mudra

PRIMARY BENEFITS

■ Produces heartwarming and grounding sensations

SIGNIFICANCE

■ Symbolizes connection of your inner wisdom or heart to the earth

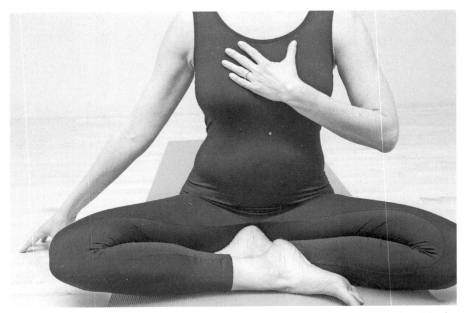

Heart Centering *Mudra*

MUDRA INSTRUCTIONS

1. Place your left palm over your heart.

2. Lightly touch the earth with your right fingertips to your right side. When seated in a chair, direct your right fingers toward the earth.

3. Enjoy Heart Centering *Mudra* for several breaths.

Ksepana Mudra

PRIMARY BENEFITS

■ Stimulates elimination

■ Encourages release of toxins, negative thoughts and emotions

SIGNIFICANCE

■ Directs negative energy away from you

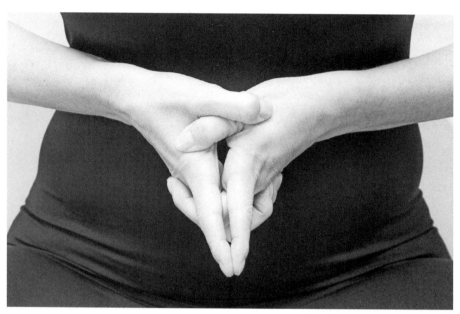

Ksepana Mudra

MUDRA INSTRUCTIONS

1. Interlace your pinky, ring, and middle fingers at the webbing.

2. Clasp your hands like you are shaking hands with yourself. Then extend your index fingers with fingertips touching.

3. Cross your left thumb over your right thumb at the lowest knuckle.

4. Create space between palms and index fingers.

5. Point your fingers toward the earth.

6. Enjoy *Ksepana Mudra*. Inhale and exhale deeply for several breaths for a maximum of 2 minutes.

≪≫ *Padma Mudra*

PRIMARY BENEFITS

▨ Promotes compassion

▨ Opens heart to positive feelings

▨ Supports cardio, respiratory, and immune systems

SIGNIFICANCE

▨ Symbolizes pure heart and open mind

▨ Represents lotus flower

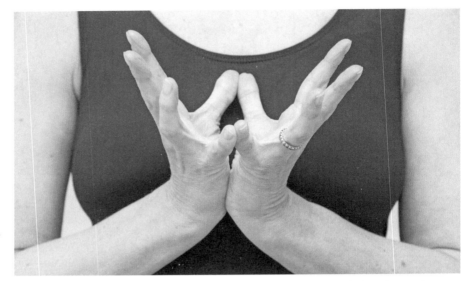

Padma Mudra (Lotus *Mudra*) with petals open

MUDRA INSTRUCTIONS

1. Join your hands in three places: at the heel of your palms; and at the fingertips of the pinky fingers and thumbs.
2. Spread the middle three fingers apart to form a blossoming flower.
3. Place the *mudra* in front of your heart.
4. Enjoy *Padma Mudra* for several breaths.

Pala Mudra

PRIMARY BENEFITS

■ Reduces stress and anxiety

■ Increases sense of security and trust

SIGNIFICANCE

■ Represents monk's begging bowl

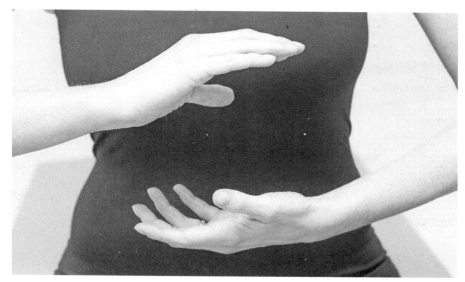

Pala Mudra

MUDRA INSTRUCTIONS

1. Cup each hand, and place your left hand a few inches below your navel, palm facing skyward.
2. Place your cupped right hand a few inches above your navel, palm facing toward the earth. Your palms are facing each other.
3. Enjoy *Pala Mudra* for several breaths.

Prithvi Mudra

PRIMARY BENEFITS

■ Reduces physical weakness, fatigue, and instability

■ Grounds or centers energy toward earth

SIGNIFICANCE

■ Represents strong roots

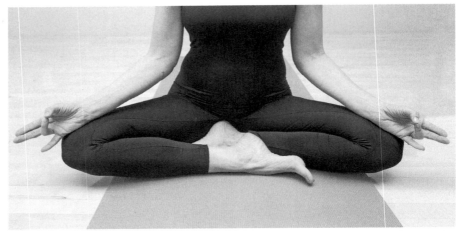

Prithvi Mudra

MUDRA INSTRUCTIONS

1. Join the ring finger and thumb on both hands while opening and extending the index, middle and pinky fingers away from the palms.

2. Rest the backs of your hands on your knees or thighs, with palms skyward.

3. Enjoy *Prithvi Mudra* for several breaths, OR while meditating.

Vyana Vayu Mudra

PRIMARY BENEFITS

■ Promotes healthy central nervous system (CNS)

■ Stimulates healing energy for neurological conditions such as multiple sclerosis

SIGNIFICANCE

■ Symbolizes both earth and air elements

■ Represents communication and clear energy flow throughout body

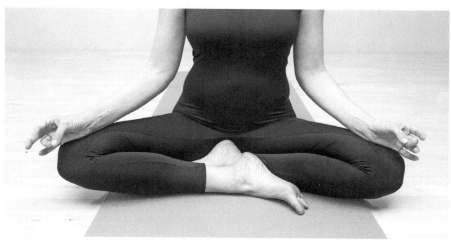

Vyana Vayu Mudra

MUDRA INSTRUCTIONS

1. On the right hand join the thumb and ring finger together, and on the left hand, join the thumb and middle finger together.

2. Rest the backs of your hands on your knees or thighs, with the palms facing downward OR skyward.

3. Enjoy *Vyana Vayu Mudra* for several breaths, or while meditating. This is sometimes called the MS *Mudra*.

ADAPTATION TO *VYANA VAYU MUDRA*

• Practice with palms facing toward the earth to decrease sensations such as tingling, OR temperature change, OR when new to this *mudra*. This will have a more calming effect.

CHAPTER 9

There are a thousand ways to kneel and kiss the earth.

RUMI

Playful, Empowering, and Healing Sequences

"Playful, Empowering, and Healing Sequences" bring the yoga moves in this book together. Yoga Moves sequences for a particular time of day, place, or focus are divided into categories.

• Yoga Moves Transition Sequences **T**

• Yoga Moves in a Chair Sequences **C**

• Yoga Moves on the Earth Sequences **E**

• Yoga Moves Mixed Sequences **M**

A daily dose of yoga combined with a breathing practice lubricates your joints, moves your spine, opens your hips and shoulders, and improves posture and balance. In addition, resting in the closing pose allows your body to absorb the benefits of practice and calms the nervous system. Each sequence includes some or all of the following:

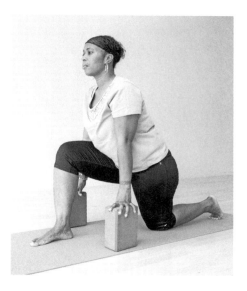

• Breathing practice
• Warm Up, Tune Up, and Loosen Up Moves
• Centering poses
• Side bends
• Core builders
• Balance poses
• Twists
• Backbends
• Forward bends
• Hip openers
• Restorative poses
• Hand *Mudras*

Sequences contain a prompting photo with a corresponding page number for each step. There you can find more detailed instructions, adaptations, and variations for the recommended sequence pose. The times to complete each sequence are estimated and vary depending upon your practice. For asymmetrical poses, remember to practice the instructions using both left and right sides of your body. Optional hand *mudras* are best practiced in a comfortable seated posture at the beginning or end of a sequence.

Playful, Empowering, and Healing Sequences

Videos of selected sequences are available on yogamovesms.org.

On any given day, select a sequence that complements your energy, mood, mind and body. Different sequences may feature different energetic qualities. They may provide a practice that is awakening, balancing, calming, focusing, invigorating, meditative, refreshing, restorative, rhythmic, strengthening, stretching, cooling, or warming.

Once you are comfortable with the sequences provided, mix and match them, and explore your own creativity by forming your own sequences. Just as you may skip a pose, you may add a pose to a sequence based on your needs. Sequences can be practiced alone or together with others.

Seek medical advice to be sure you are physically capable of performing these sequences safely.

INSTRUCTIONS FOR SEQUENCE PRACTICE

1. Choose a sequence.
2. Note and tab the pages and variations that you would like to have handy for your practice, and read the instructions for each step.
3. Place your yoga mat where needed, either in the center of the room, or near a wall. Gather and set up any required props near your yoga mat.
4. For easy reference, place the book or a photocopy of your selected sequence next to your mat. Alternatively, ask a buddy to read the instructions to you.
5. Set the tone for your practice with a personal intention, poem, or dedication.
6. Practice the Complete Yoga Breath for 3 to 5 breaths before beginning each sequence, and consciously breathe throughout the steps.
7. Enjoy the final resting pose. It may be helpful to set a timer for how long you wish to rest.
8. End your practice with a brief moment of gratitude. This provides transition to the next phase of your day.
9. *Namaste.* I honor the light within you.

Yoga Moves Transition Sequences

Safe Landing: From a Chair to the Earth Sequence

PRIMARY BENEFITS

▪ Enables yoga practice on the earth

▪ Enables play with children and pets on earth

PRECAUTIONS

▪ Dizziness

▪ Neck, hand, wrist, elbow, shoulder, ankle, knee, or hip pain, injury, or condition

▪ Practice Safe Landing variations with a qualified assistant until you are confident and competent to transfer from a chair to the earth without assistance

PROPS

▪ Yoga mat

▪ Chair(s)

▪ Wall

▪ Blanket(s)

▪ Yoga buddy

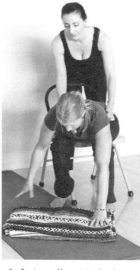

Safe Landing Variation 1: Step 1, 2, 3 and 4

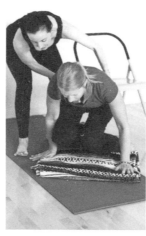

Safe Landing Variation 1: Step 5

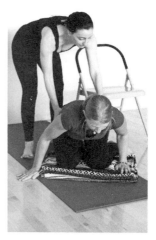

Safe Landing Variation 1: Step 6

VARIATION 1

1. Place a mat on your preferred side of a chair.

2. Place any blankets or padding on your mat where your knees and hands will land.

3. Move your hips to the edge of the chair.

4. Bend at your hips, and reach your hands toward the earth.

5. Walk your hands forward when they touch the earth, and slowly lift your hips off of the chair.

6. Lower onto your knees with care and celebrate your safe landing.

7. Center yourself before you move toward your intended pose (for example, Stick Pose, Table Pose, or Child's Pose).

Safe Landing: From a Chair to the Earth Sequence

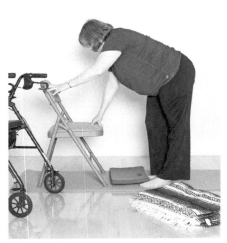

Safe Landing
Variation 2: Steps 1, 2 and 3

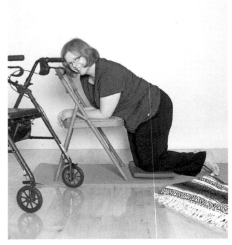

Safe Landing
Variation 2: Steps 4 and 5

VARIATION 2

1. Stand and face a chair, preferably placed against a wall for stability.

2. Place your hands on the chair.

3. Walk your feet back until you are in an "L" position, similar to Wall Dog Pose with a chair (see page 307 for instructions).

4. Lower your knees to the mat with care and celebrate a safe landing.

5. Center yourself before you move to your intended pose (for example, Stick Pose, Table Pose, or Child's Pose).

T *Lift Off: From the Earth to a Chair or Standing Sequence*

PRIMARY BENEFITS

■ Enables yoga practice on the earth

■ Enables play with children and pets on earth

PRECAUTIONS

■ Dizziness

■ Neck, hand, wrist, elbow, shoulder, ankle, knee, or hip pain, injury, or condition

■ Practice Lift Off variations with a qualified assisstant until you are confident and competent to transfer from the earth to a chair or standing without assistance.

PROPS

■ Yoga mat

■ Chair(s)

■ Wall

■ Yoga buddy

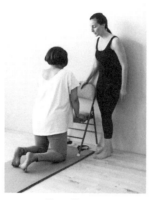

Lift Off Variation 1:
Steps 1 and 2

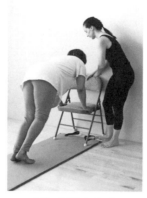

Lift Off Variation 1:
Step 3

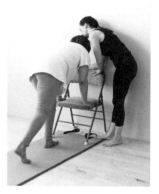

Lift Off Variation 1:
Step 4

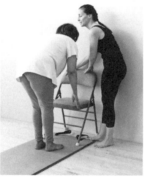

Lift Off Variation 1:
Step 5

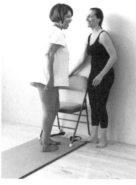

Lift Off Variation 1:
Steps 5 and 6

VARIATION 1

1. Place the back of a chair against the wall before you lower to the earth.

2. Position yourself facing the chair and stand on your knees. Place your palms on the chair seat.

3. Lift your hips and knees together into an "L" position, similar to Wall Dog Pose with a chair (see page 307 for instructions).

4. Step one foot forward.

5. Step the other foot forward as you slowly rise to a standing position.

6. Enjoy 3 to 5 breaths and celebrate that you have safely lifted off the earth.

Lift Off: From the Earth to a Chair or Standing Sequence

VARIATION 2

1. Place a chair against the wall before you lower down to the earth.

2. Face the chair standing on your knees. Place your hands on the sides of the seat.

3. Step your right foot forward while holding onto the chair.

4. Lift your left knee.

5. Step your left foot to meet your right foot as you rise to an "L" position, similar to Wall Dog Pose with a chair (see page 307 for instructions).

6. Take a seat in the chair or rise to a standing position.

7. Enjoy 3 to 5 breaths and celebrate that you have safely lifted off the earth.

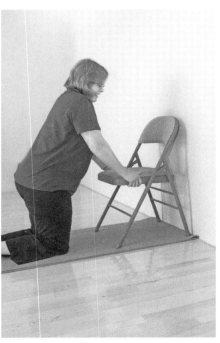

Lift Off Variation 2:
Steps 1 and 2

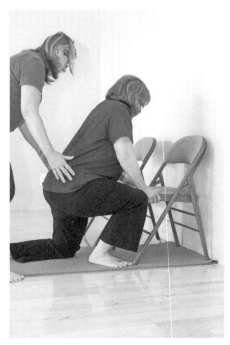

Lift Off Variation 2:
Steps 3 and 4

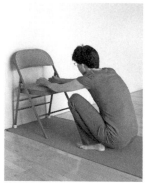
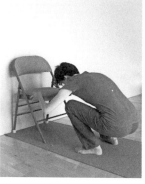
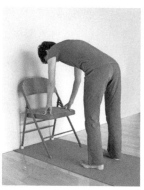

Lift Off Variation 3: Steps 1 and 2   Lift Off Variation 3: Steps 3 and 4   Lift Off Variation 3: Steps 5 and 6

VARIATION 3

Attempt this transition only if you are confident in Yoga Squat Pose

1. Place the back of a chair against the wall before you lower to the earth.

2. Face the chair seat in Yoga Squat Pose (see page 321 for instructions).

3. Place your hands on the chair seat.

4. Lift your hips.

5. Straighten your knees as you rise into an "L" position, similar to Wall Dog Pose with a chair (see page 307 for instructions).

6. Enjoy 3 to 5 breaths and celebrate that you have safely lifted off the earth.

Get Moving Basic Chair Sequence

ENERGETIC QUALITIES: strengthening, stretching, invigorating

TIME ESTIMATE: 10 to 15 minutes

PROPS: yoga mat, chair, block, yoga strap, blanket

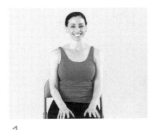

1   p222

Mountain Pose in a Chair

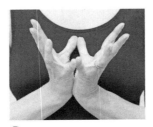

2   p222

Padma Mudra

(p.334, optional)

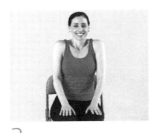

3   p67

Shoulder Circles

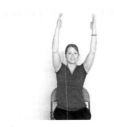

4   p68

Arm Lift

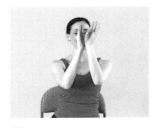

5   p83

Candle Flame Wrist Release

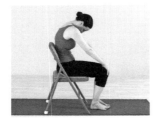

6   p148

Cat Pose in a Chair

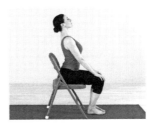

7   p148

Cow Pose in a Chair

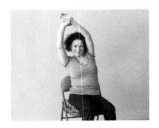

8   p103

Side Bend in a Chair

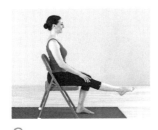

9   p115

Ankle Circles

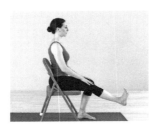

10   p116

Flex

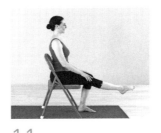

11   p116

Point

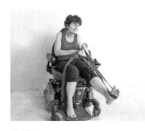

12   p210

Leg Stretch Pose in a Chair

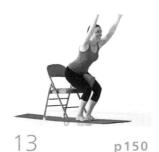

13   p150

Chair Pose

14

Practice the following Steps 15,16, &17 together on the right side. Then practice them together on the left side.

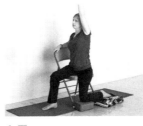

15   p160

Crescent Pose in a Chair

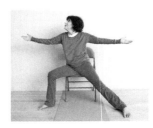

16   p312

Warrior 2 Pose in a Chair

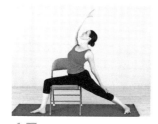

17   p312

**Reverse Warrior Pose
in a chair**

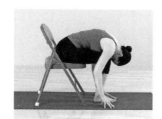

18   p185

**Forward Fold Pose
in a chair**

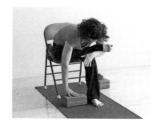

19   p130

 # 4 Pose in a chair

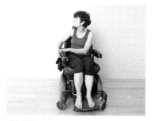

20   p271

**Spinal Twist Pose
in a chair**

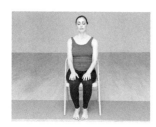

21   p238

**Relaxation Pose
in a chair**

C *It Takes Two or (more) to Tango Chair Sequence*

ENERGETIC QUALITIES: stretching, strengthening, balancing, refreshing

TIME ESTIMATE: 5 to 10 minutes

PROPS: 3 chairs, yoga strap, blanket(s)

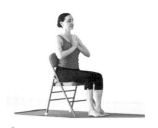

1   p222

Mountain Pose in a Chair with *Anjali Mudra* (p.326, optional)

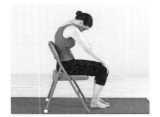

2   p148

Cat Pose in a Chair

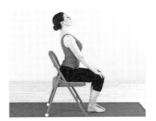

3   p148

Cow Pose in a Chair

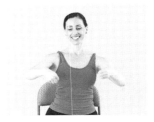

4   p82

Wrist Circles

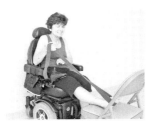

5   p210

Leg Stretch Pose in a Chair

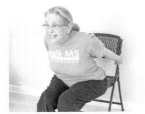

6   p79

Seated Backbend

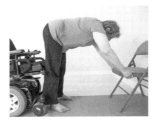

7   p305

Wall Dog Pose with 2 chairs

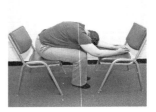

8   p153

Child's Pose with 2 chairs

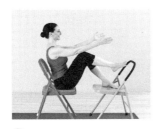

9   p133

Boat Pose with 2 chairs

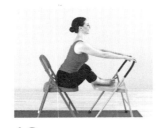

10   p140

Butterfly Pose with 2 chairs

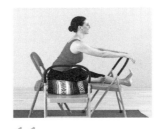

11   p293

Tree Pose with 3 chairs

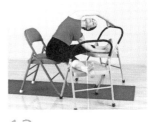

12   p316

Wide Angle Forward Fold Pose with 3 chairs and a side bend

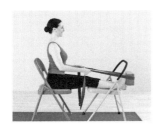

13   p276

Stick Pose with 2 chairs

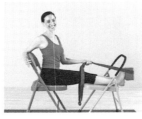

14   p276

Stick Pose with 2 chairs in a twist

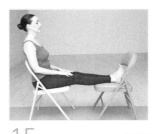

15   p238

Relaxation Pose with 2 chairs

C *Seated Sun Salutations Sequence*

ENERGETIC QUALITIES: invigorating, stretching, strengthening, rhythmic

TIME ESTIMATE: 15 to 20 minutes

PROPS: yoga mat, chair

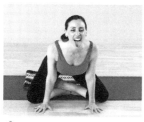

1   p35
Lion's Breath

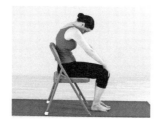

2   p148
Cat Pose in a Chair

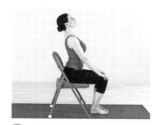

3   p148
Cow Pose in a Chair

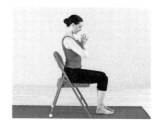

4   p222
Sun Salutation begins here: *Anjali Mudra*
(p.326, optional)

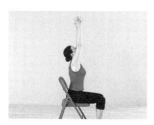

5   p68
Arms Circle Skyward

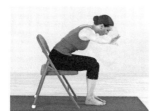

6   p185
Forward Fold Pose in a Chair

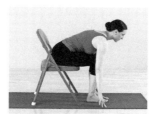

7
Extended spine and forward gaze

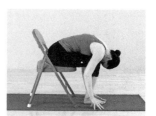

8   p185
Forward Fold Pose in a Chair

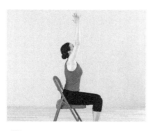

9   p68
Arms Circle Skyward

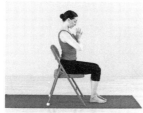

10   p222
Anjali Mudra
(p.326, optional)

11

Repeat Sun Salutation, steps 4 to 10, 3 more times

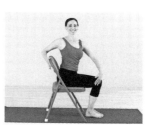

12   p271
Spinal Twist Pose in a chair

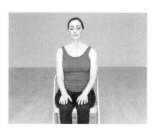

13   p238
Relaxation Pose in a chair

C *Playing Footsie Sequence*

ENERGETIC QUALITIES: rhythmic, calming, refreshing

TIME ESTIMATE: 10 minutes

PROPS: yoga mat, chair, tennis ball, box

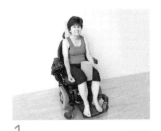

1   p222

Mountain Pose in a Chair

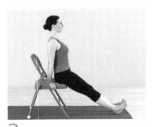

2   p210

Leg Stretch Pose in a Chair

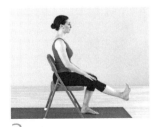

3   p116

Flex

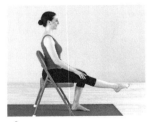

4   p116

Point

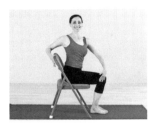

5   p271

Spinal Twist Pose in a chair

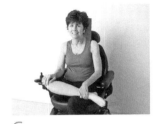

6   p130

#4 Pose in a chair

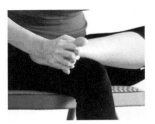

7   p121

Yoga Handshake

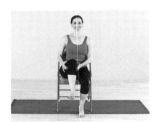

8   p123

Walking While Seated

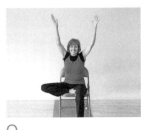

9   p296

Tree Pose in a chair

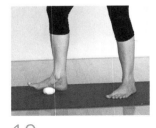

10   p120

Pressure Point Foot Massage

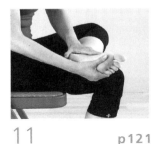

11   p121

Foot Massage

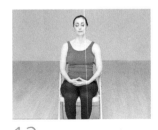

12   p238

Relaxation Pose in a chair with *Dhyana Mudra* *(p.329, optional)*

C *Opening the Heart Sequence*

ENERGETIC QUALITIES: stretching, strengthening, invigorating, refreshing

TIME ESTIMATE: 10 to 15 minutes

PROPS: yoga mat, chair, wall, table, blanket, yoga strap

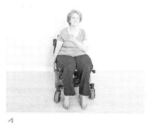

1   p222

Mountain Pose in a Chair, Heart Centering *Mudra* *(p.332, optional)*

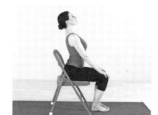

2   p148

Cat Pose in a Chair

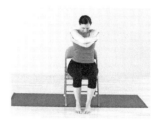

3   p148

Cow Pose in a Chair

4

Yoga Hug

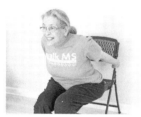

5   p79

Backbend in a Chair

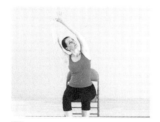

7   p101

Side Bend in a chair

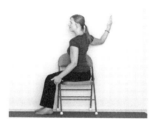

8   p74

Shoulder Opener at the Wall

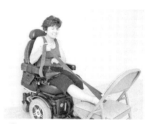

6   p210

Leg Stretch Pose in a Chair

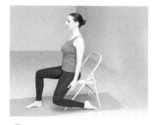

9   p160

Crescent Pose in a Chair

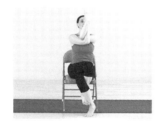

10   p172

Eagle Pose in a Chair

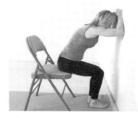

11   p198

Headstand Pose in a chair

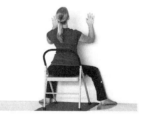

12   p158

Cobra Pose in a Chair at the Wall

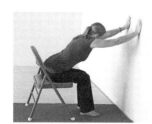

13   p305

Wall Dog Pose in a chair

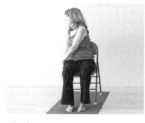

14   p271

Spinal Twist Pose in a Chair

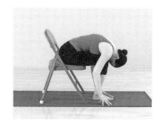

15   p185

Forward Fold Pose in a Chair

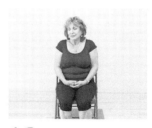

16   p238

Relaxation Pose in a chair

C Legs Gone Restless, Rigid and Spastic Sequence

ENERGETIC QUALITIES: stretching, calming

TIME ESTIMATE: 10 to 15 minutes

PROPS: yoga mat, 1 to 2 chairs, yoga strap, blanket

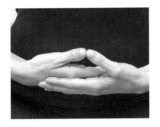

1   p222
Mountain Pose in a Chair, *Dhyana Mudra* *(p.329, optional)*

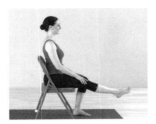

2   p115
Ankle Circles

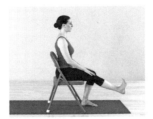

3   p116
Flex

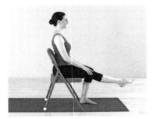

4   p116
Point

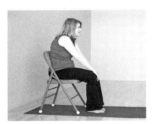

5   p148
Cat Pose in a Chair

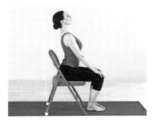

6   p148
Cow Pose in a Chair

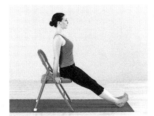

7   p210
Leg Stretch Pose in a Chair with Flexed Toes

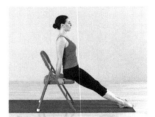

8   p210
Leg Stretch Pose in Chair with Pointed Toes

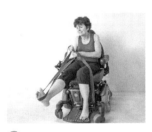

9   p210
Leg Stretch Pose in a chair with strap

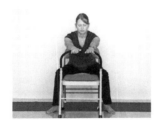

10   p187
Goddess Pose with 2 Chairs

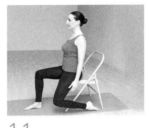

11   p160
Crescent Pose in a Chair

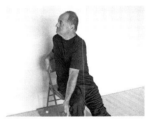

12   p255
Sage Twist Pose in a chair

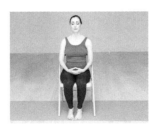

13   p238
Relaxation Pose in a chair

C Computer Break Sequence

ENERGETIC QUALITIES: stretching, refreshing, focusing, calming

TIME ESTIMATE: 10 minutes

PROPS: chair, yoga strap, table top or desk

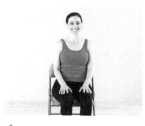

1 p222
Mountain Pose in a Chair

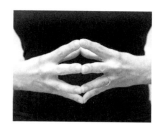

2 p222
Hakini Mudra
(p.331, optional)

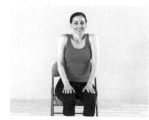

3 p67
Shoulder Circles

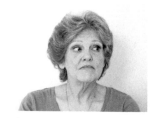

4 p65
Yoga Moves Your Eyes

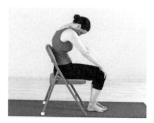

5 p148
Cat Pose in a Chair

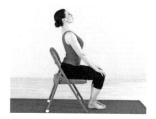

6 p148
Cow Pose in a Chair

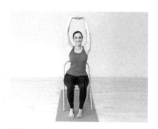

7 p69
Fingers interlaced

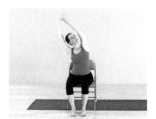

8 p101
Side Bend in a Chair with thumbs interlaced

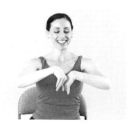

9 p83
Candle Flame Wrist Release

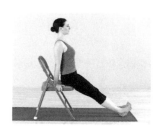

10 p210
Leg Stretch Pose in a Chair

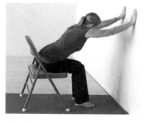

11 p305
Wall Dog Pose in a chair

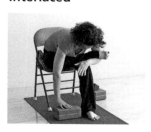

12 p130
#4 Pose in a chair

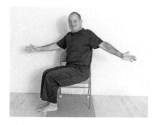

13 p271
Spinal Twist Pose in a Chair

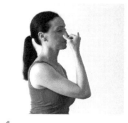

14 p32
Alternate Nostril Breath

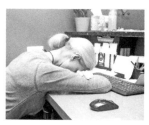

15 p248
Restorative Forward Fold Pose in a chair

Practice 1 to 3 Mindful Meditation minutes

p24

C Preparing to Transfer In and Out of Car Sequence

ENERGETIC QUALITIES: stretching, strengthening, rhythmic

TIME ESTIMATE: 10 to 15 minutes

PROPS: yoga mat, chairs, yoga strap, blanket

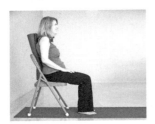

1   p222

Mountain Pose in a Chair

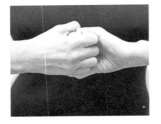

2   p222

Ganesha Mudra
(p.330, optional)

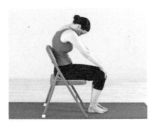

3   p148

Cat Pose in a Chair

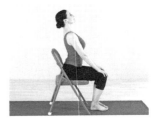

4   p148

Cow Pose in a Chair

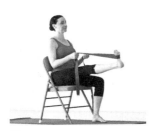

5   p210

Leg Stretch Pose in a Chair

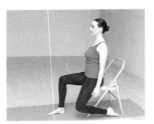

6   p160

Crescent Pose in a Chair

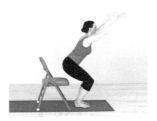

7   p150

Chair Pose

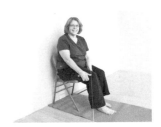

8   p123

Walking While Seated

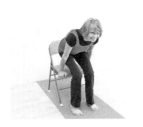

9   p258

Scale Pose in a chair

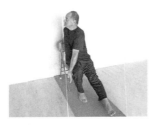

10   p255

Sage Twist Pose in a Chair

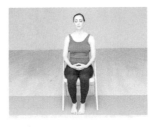

11   p238

Relaxation Pose in a chair

Reclining Wall Sequence

ENERGETIC QUALITIES: stretching, strengthening, restorative

TIME ESTIMATE: 20 to 25 minutes

PROPS: yoga mat, wall, blanket, yoga strap
Place short end of mat next to wall

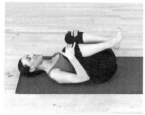

1   p106

Spinal Massage
(place head an arm's distance from wall)

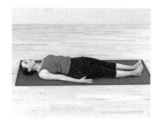

2   p224

Pelvic Tilt Pose

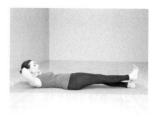

3   p221

Mountain Pose on the Earth

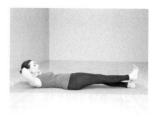

4   p90

Head and Leg Lift

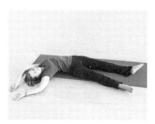

5   p104

Side Bend on the earth

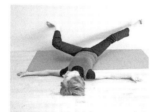

6   p308

Warrior 2 Pose on the earth *(you may keep mat perpendicular to wall)*

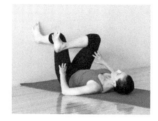

7   p130

#4 Pose at the wall Pose

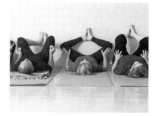

8   p212

Legs Up the Wall Pose with "butterfly" legs

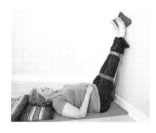

9   p212

Legs Up the Wall Pose

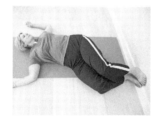

10   p274

Spinal Twist Pose Reclining
(press feet into wall)

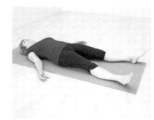

11   p238

Relaxation Pose

E Kiss the Earth Sequence

ENERGETIC QUALITIES: stretching, strengthening, refreshing

TIME ESTIMATE: 20 minutes

PROPS: yoga mat, block, yoga strap, blanket

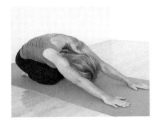

1 p153
Child's Pose

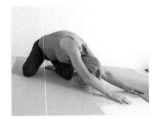

2 p153
Child's Pose side stretch

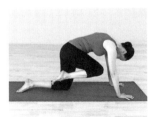

3 p283
Table Pose with Knee to Chest

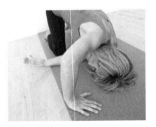

4 p291
Thread the Needle Pose

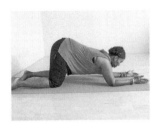

5 p280
Table Pose on forearms

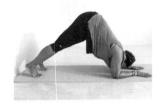

6 p168
Dolphin Dog Pose

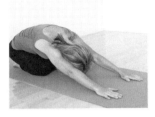

7 p153
Child's Pose

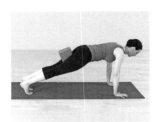

8 p230
Plank Pose

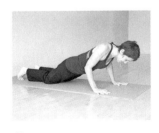

9 p230
Yoga Push-Up

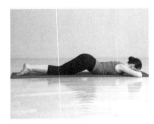

10 p205
Inchworm Pose

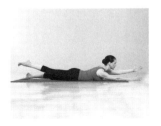

11 p218
Locust Pose

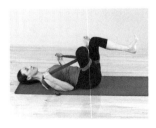

12 p130
#4 Pose

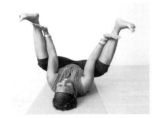

13 p196
Happy Baby Pose

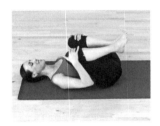

14 p106
Spinal Massage

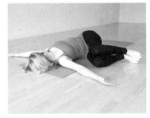

15 p274
Spinal Twist Pose Reclining

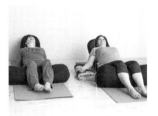

16 p238
Relaxation Pose

E *Float Your Boat Core Building Sequence*

ENERGETIC QUALITIES: stretching, strengthening, invigorating

TIME ESTIMATE: 15 minutes

PROPS: yoga mat, block, yoga strap, blanket, chair

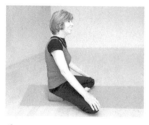

1 p175
Easy Pose

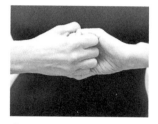

2 p175
Ganesha Mudra
(p.330, optional)

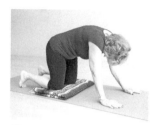

3 p146
Cat and Cow Poses

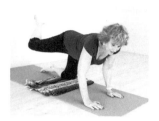

4 p285
**Table Pose
with Knee Circles**

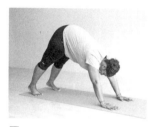

5 p170
**Downward Facing
Dog Pose**

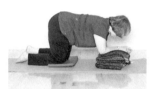

6 p280
**Table Pose
on forearms**

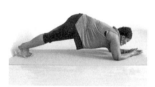

7 p230
**Plank Pose
on forearms**

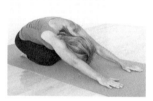

8 p153
Child's Pose

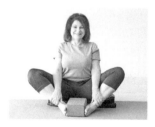

9 p140
Butterfly Pose

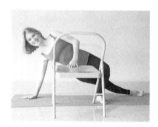

10 p260
Side Plank Pose

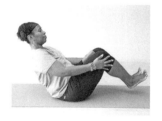

11 p133
Boat Pose

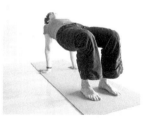

12 p286
Table Pose in Reverse

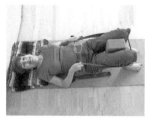

13 p137
Bridge Pose

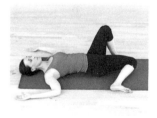

14 p274
**Windshield
Wiper Pose**

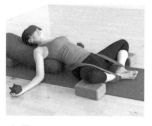

15 p245
**Restorative
Butterfly Pose**

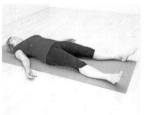

16 p238
Relaxation Pose
(optional)

E Finding Balance Sequence

ENERGETIC QUALITIES: stretching, strengthening, invigorating, balancing

TIME ESTIMATE: 15 to 20 minutes

PROPS: yoga mat, wall, blocks, blanket

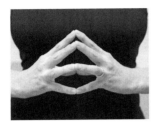

1   p175

Easy Pose with
Hakini Mudra
(p.331, optional)

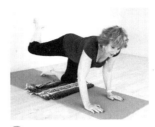

2   p175

Alternate Nostril Breath, p 32

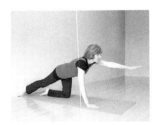

3   p285

Table Pose with Knee Circles

4   p268

Spinal Balance Pose

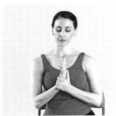

5   p81

Julie's Hand and Wrist Release

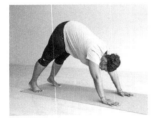

6   p170

Downward Facing Dog Pose

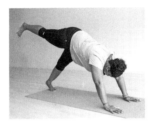

7   p170

3-Legged Downward Facing Dog Pose

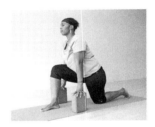

8   p162

Crescent Kneeling Lunge Pose

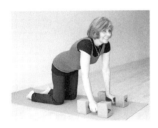

9   p280

Table Pose

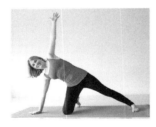

10   p263

Gate Pose

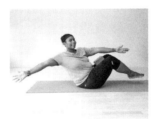

11   p133

Boat Pose with a twist

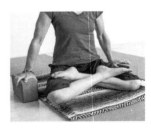

12   p258

Scale Pose

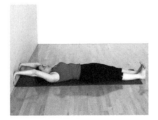

13   p194

Handstand Pose on the Earth

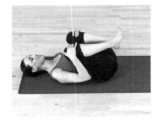

14   p106

Juicy Hips Spinal Massage

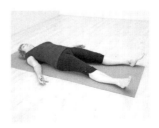

15   p238

Relaxation Pose

ⓔ *Open Your Heart Sequence*

ENERGETIC QUALITIES: stretching, strengthening, refreshing, restorative

TIME ESTIMATE: 20 minutes

PROPS: yoga mat, chair, wall, blocks, yoga strap, 1 to 2 blanket(s), bolster

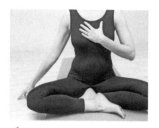

1   p175

Easy Pose with Heart Centering *Mudra*

(p.332, optional)

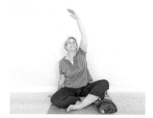

2   p102

Side Bend in Easy Pose

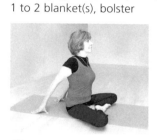

3   p175

Easy Pose with backbend

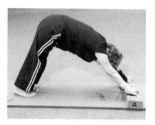

4   p170

Downward Facing Dog Pose

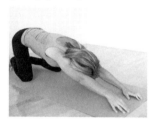

5   p234

Puppy Pose

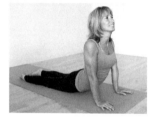

6   p156

Cobra Pose

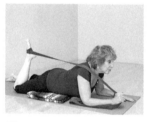

7   p288

Thigh Stretch Pose on the Earth

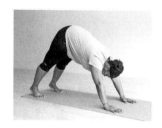

8   p170

Downward Facing Dog Pose

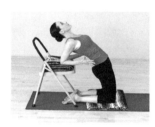

9   p144

Camel Pose

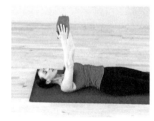

10   p91

Arm Lift

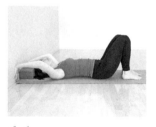

11   p198

Headstand Pose on the Earth

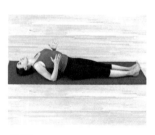

12   p64

Fish Pose

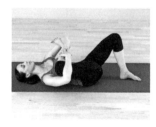

13   p229

Rock-The-Baby Pose

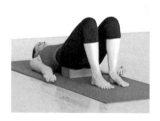

14   p241

Restorative Backbend with Block Variation

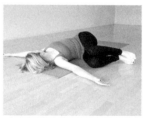

15   p274

Spinal Twist Pose Reclining

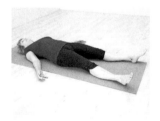

16   p238

Relaxation Pose

E Legs Gone Restless, Rigid and Spastic Sequence

ENERGETIC QUALITIES: stretching, strengthening, invigorating, balancing

TIME ESTIMATE: 15 to 20 minutes

PROPS: yoga mat, wall, 2 blocks, yoga strap

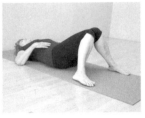

1   p28
Constructive Rest Pose with Complete Yoga Breath

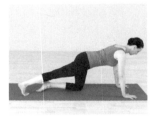

2   p284
Table Pose with Leg Extended on Earth
(roll heel forward and backward)

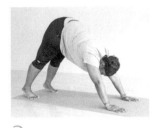

3   p170
Downward Facing Dog Pose

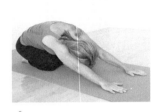

4   p153
Child's Pose

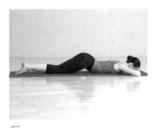

5   p205
Inchworm Pose

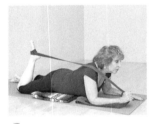

6   p288
Thigh Stretch Pose on the Earth

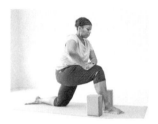

7   p162
Crescent Kneeling Lunge Pose

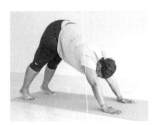

8   p170
Downward Facing Dog Pose

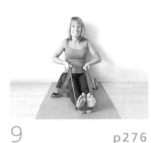

9   p276
Stick Pose

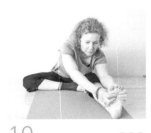

10   p296
Tree Pose Seated on the Earth

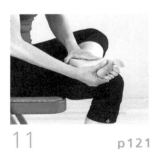

11   p121
Foot Massage

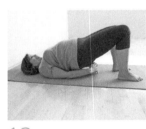

12   p137
Bridge Pose

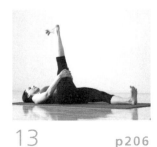

13   p206
Leg Stretch Pose on the Back

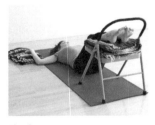

14   p212
Legs on the Chair Pose

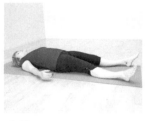

15   p238
Relaxation Pose

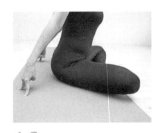

16   p175
Easy Pose, *Bhu Mudra*
(p.327, optional)

E *As Good as a Nap, Restore and Renew Sequence*

ENERGETIC QUALITIES: stretching, calming, restorative, refreshing

TIME ESTIMATE: 20 minutes to 1 hour.

PROPS: yoga mat, wall, block, yoga strap, blanket(s), bolster

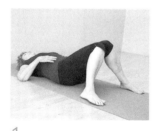

1   p28

**Constructive
Rest Pose**

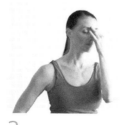

2   p32

**Alternate Nostril
Breath** *(optional: on the
earth variation)*

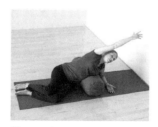

3   p105

**Side Bend over
bolster**

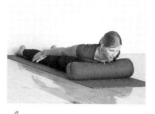

4   p156

**Cobra Pose
with bolster**

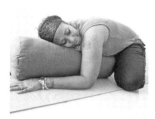

5   p153

**Child's Pose
with bolster**

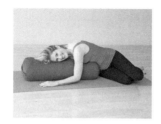

6   p249

**Restorative Twist
Pose over bolster**

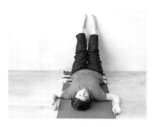

7   p212

**Legs Up the Wall
Pose**

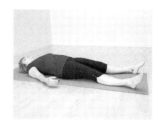

8   p238

Relaxation Pose

*Remain in each restorative pose from 3 to 20 minutes.
You may choose 1 or all poses for a "pick me up".*

E *Time to Go to Bed, Sleepy Head Sequence*

ENERGETIC QUALITIES: stretching, restorative, calming

TIME ESTIMATE: 15 to 1 hour

PROPS: yoga mat, yoga strap, blanket, bolster, favorite cream or oil for feet, guided imagery, or yoga *nidra*

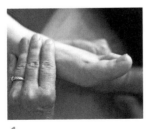

1   p121

Foot Massage

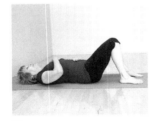

2   p137

Bridge Prep Pose

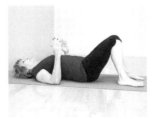

3   p224

Pelvic Tilt Pose

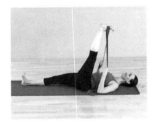

4   p206

Leg Stretch Pose on the Back

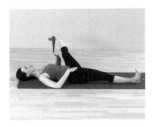

5   p206

Leg Stretch Pose on the Back (leg to the side)

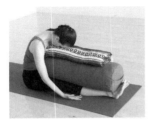

6   p247

Restorative Forward Fold Pose

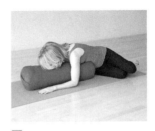

7   p249

Restorative Twist Pose with bolster

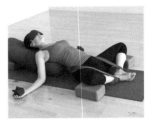

8   p245

Restorative Butterfly Pose

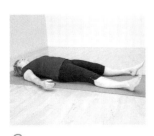

9   p238

Relaxation Pose and Guided Imagery or Body Scan *(p.26)*

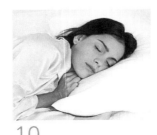

10

Sweet Dreams

Sequence can be practiced in bed or on the earth. Keep yoga strap near bedside in case of restless legs, leg cramps, or spasms during sleep.

Yoga Moves Mixed Sequences

Get Out of Bed, Sleepy Head

ENERGETIC QUALITIES: stretching, strengthening, awakening

TIME ESTIMATE: 10 TO 15 minutes

PROPS: bed, comfortable meditation seat

NOTE: Steps 1 to 12 can be practiced while in bed

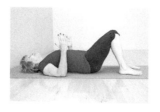

1 p137

Bridge Prep Pose

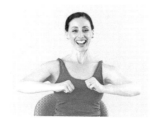

2 p82

Wrist Circles

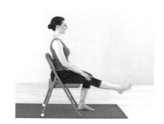

3 p115

Ankle Circles

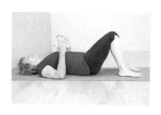

4 p224

Pelvic Tilt Pose

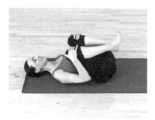

5 p106

Juicy Hips

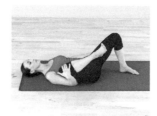

6 p106

Knee Circles

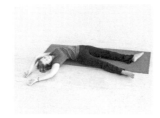

7 p104

Side Bend on the earth

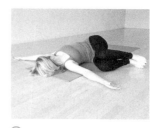

8 p274

Spinal Twist Pose Reclining

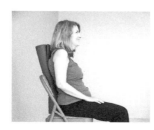

9 p222

Mountain Pose in a Chair *(on side of bed)*

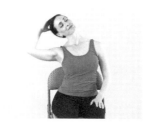

10 p61

Scalene Stretch

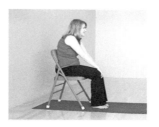

11 p148

Cat Pose in a Chair

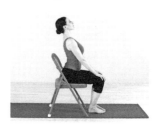

12 p148

Cow Pose in a Chair

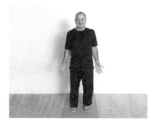

13 p220

Mountain Pose

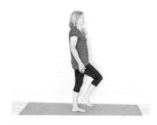

14 p126

Compassionate Steps to the kitchen

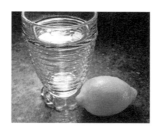

15

Enjoy warm lemon water

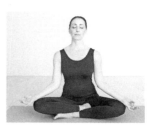

16 p24

Morning Meditation

Ⓜ Get Up! Stand Up! Get Down! Basic Mixed Sequence

ENERGETIC QUALITIES: stretching, strengthening, refreshing

TIME ESTIMATE: 30 to 40 minutes

PROPS: yoga mat, chair, wall, blankets, yoga strap

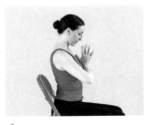

1   p222
Mountain Pose in a Chair, *Anjali Mudra* (p.326, optional)

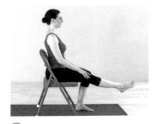

2   p82
Wrist Circles

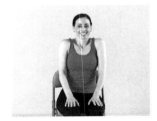

3   p115
Ankle Circles

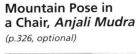

4   p67
Shoulder Circles

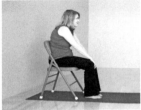

5   p148
Cat Pose in a Chair

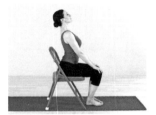

6   p148
Cow Pose in a Chair

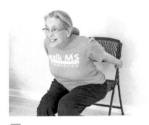

7   p79
Backbend in a chair

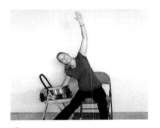

8   p300
Triangle Pose in a chair

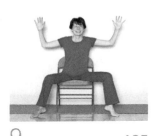

9   p187
Goddess Pose in a Chair with heels lifted

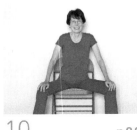

10   p98
Goddess Pose Pelvic Exercise

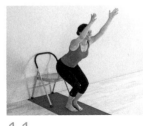

11   p150
Chair Pose

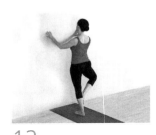

12   p243
Tree Pose at the wall

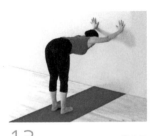

13   p305
Wall Dog Pose

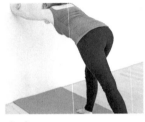

14   p236
Pyramid Pose

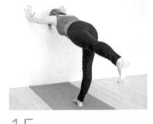

15   p314
Warrior 3 Pose

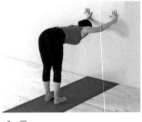

16   p305
Wall Dog Pose

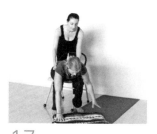

17   p341

Safe Landing: From a Chair to the Earth

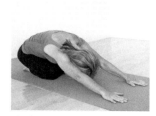

18   p153

Child's Pose

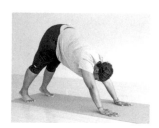

19   p170

Downward Facing Dog Pose

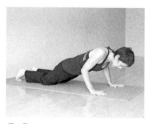

20   p233

Plank Pose on knees with yoga push-up

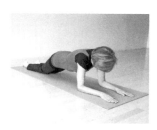

21   p94

Sphinx Core Builder

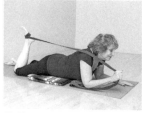

22   p288

Thigh Stretch Pose on the Earth

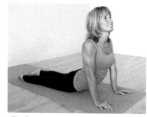

23   p156

Cobra Pose

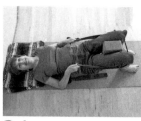

24   p137

Bridge Pose

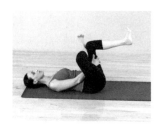

25   p130

#4 Pose

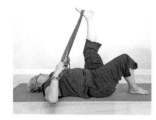

26   p206

Leg Stretch Pose on the Back

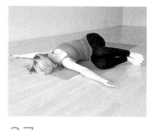

27   p274

Spinal Twist Pose Reclining

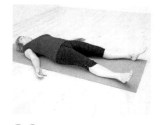

28   p238

Relaxation Pose

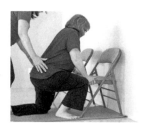

29   p343

Lift Off: From the Earth to a Chair or Standing

Ⓜ *Finding Balance*

ENERGETIC QUALITIES: stretching, strengthening, balancing, focusing

TIME ESTIMATE: 15 to 20 minutes

PROPS: yoga mat, 1 to 2 chairs, wall, block

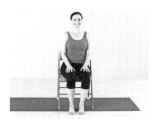

1 p222

Mountain Pose in a Chair

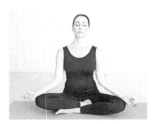

2 p222

Vyanu Vayu Mudra
(p.337, optional)

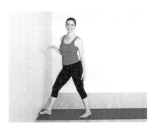

3 p118

Toe Lift at the wall

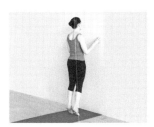

4 p119

Heel Lift

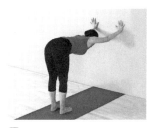

5 p305

Wall Dog Pose

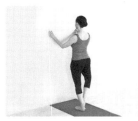

6 p293

Tree Pose

7

For ease of pose transitions, first practice all Steps 8-13 on the right side, then practice all Steps 8-13 on the left side.

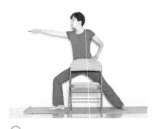

8 p308

Warrior 2 Pose

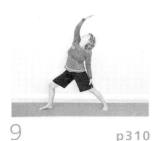

9 p310

Reverse Warrior 2 Pose

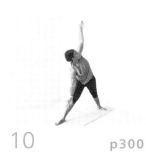

10 p300

Triangle Pose

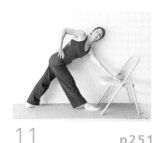

11 p251

Reverse Triangle Pose

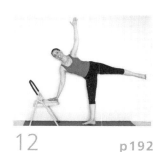

12 p192

Half Moon Pose

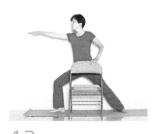

13 p308

Warrior 2 Pose

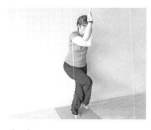

14 p173

Eagle Pose at wall

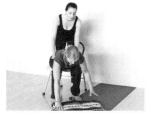

15 p341

Safe Landing: From a Chair to the Earth

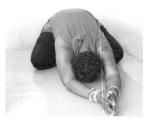

16 p153

Child's Pose

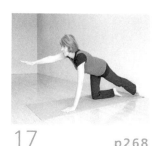

17   p268

Spinal Balance Pose

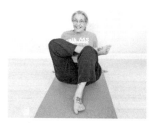

18   p130

#4 Pose

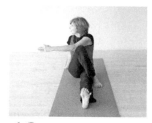

19   p255

Sage Twist Pose

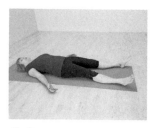

20   p238

Relaxation Pose

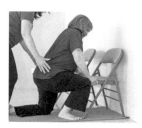

21   p343

**Lift Off: From the
Earth to a Chair or
Standing**

Sequence may be practiced with support of wall, chair, OR both a wall and a chair.

Ⓜ *Open Your Heart Sequence*

ENERGETIC QUALITIES: stretching, strengthening, invigorating, refreshing

TIME ESTIMATE: 25 to 30 minutes

PROPS: yoga mat, chair, wall, blanket

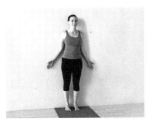

1   p220

Mountain Pose

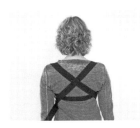

2   p78

Shlumpasana Remedy

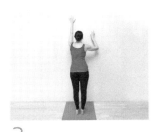

3   p77

Finger Steps

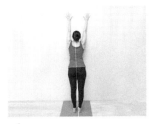

4   p76

Shower Pose

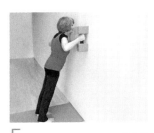

5   p233

Yoga push-up at wall

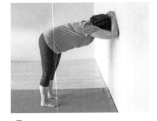

6   p198

Headstand Pose standing at wall

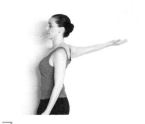

7   p73

Shoulder Opener at the Wall

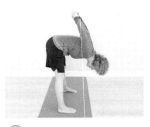

8   p320

Wide Angle Forward Fold Pose with fingers interlaced

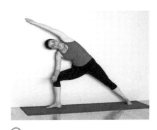

9   p177

Extended Side Angle Pose

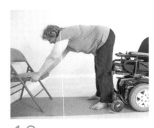

10   p305

Wall Dog Pose

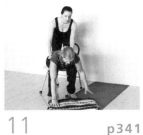

11   p341

Safe Landing: From a Chair to the Earth

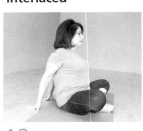

12   p140

Butterfly Pose with hands behind back

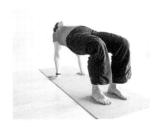

13   p286

Table Pose in Reverse

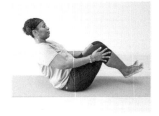

14   p133

Boat Pose

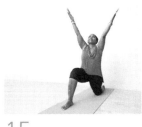

15   p162

Crescent Kneeling Lunge Pose

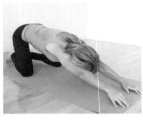

16   p234

Puppy Pose

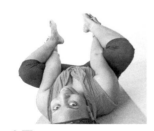

17   p196

Happy Baby Pose

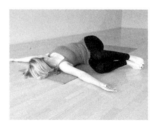

18   p274

Spinal Twist Pose Reclining

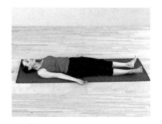

19   p238

Relaxation Pose

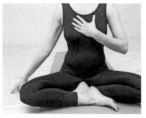

20   p175

Easy Pose with Heart Centering *Mudra* (p.332 optional)

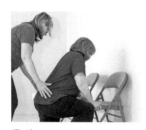

21   p343

Lift Off: From the Earth to a Chair or Standing

Sequence may be practiced with support of wall, chair, OR both a wall and a chair.

ⓜ *Mindful Steps Sequence*

ENERGETIC QUALITIES: stretching, balancing, rhythmic, refreshing, calming, meditative

TIME ESTIMATE: 20 minutes or longer, depending on walk time

PROPS: yoga mat, chair, wall, block

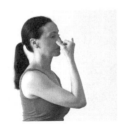

1 p32
Alternate Nostril Breath

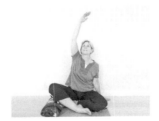

2 p102
Easy Pose with side Bend

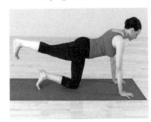

3 p280
Table Pose with leg extended and ankle circles

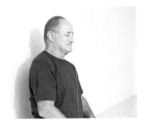

4 p202
Hero Pose

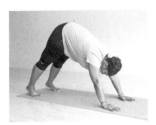

5 p170
Downward Facing Dog Pose

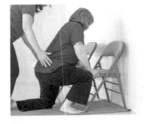

6 p343
Lift Off: From the Earth to a Chair or Standing

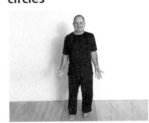

7 p115
Sole Energetics

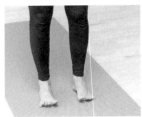

8 p118
Toe Lift

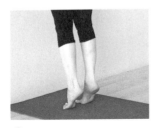

9 p119
Heel Lift

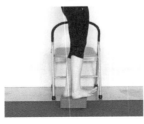

10 p113
Hip Lift

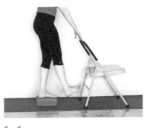

11 p112
Pendulum Swing

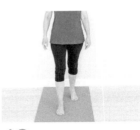

12 p124
Mindful Walking Meditation

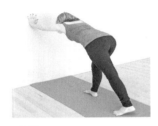

13 p236
Pyramid Pose

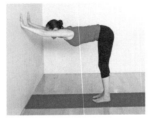

14 p305
Wall Dog Pose

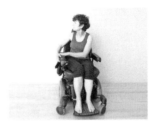

15 p271
Spinal Twist Pose in a Chair

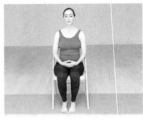

16 p238
Relaxation Pose in a chair, *Dhyana Mudra*
(p.329, optional)

Ⓜ *Loving Your Hips*

ENERGETIC QUALITIES: stretching, strengthening, grounding, restorative

TIME ESTIMATE: 25 to 30 minutes

PROPS: yoga mat, wall, blocks, blanket, bolster

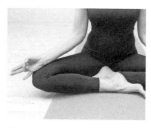

1   p175

Easy Pose, *Prithvi Mudra* (p.336, optional)

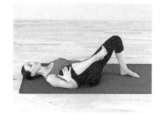

2   p106

Juicy Hips Knee Circles

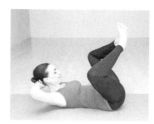

3   p93

Butterfly Core Builder

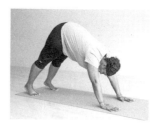

4   p170

Downward Facing Dog Pose

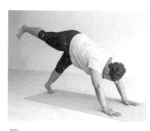

5   p170

3-Legged Downward Facing Dog Pose

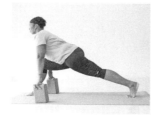

6   p166

Crescent Warrior Pose as lunge

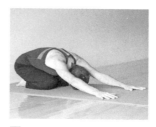

7   p153

Child's Pose

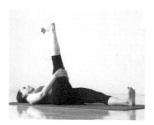

8   p206

Leg Stretch Pose on the Back

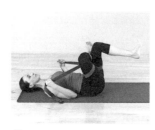

9   p130

#4 Pose

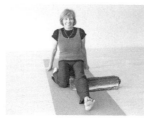

10   p202

Half Hero Pose

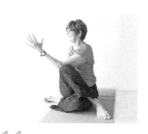

11   p189

Half Lord of the Fishes Pose

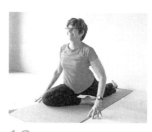

12   p227

Pigeon Pose

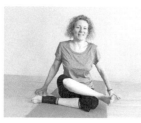

13   p180

Firelog Pose

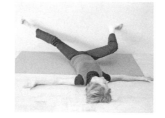

14   p308

Warrior 2 Pose at the wall

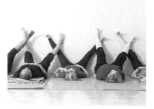

15   p212

Legs Up the Wall Pose in a "V"

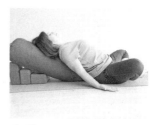

16   p245

Restorative Butterfly Pose

Ⓜ *Computer Break Sequence*

ENERGETIC QUALITIES: stretching, strengthening, refreshing

TIME ESTIMATE: 15 to 20 minutes

PROPS: yoga mat, chair, wall, table, block, yoga strap

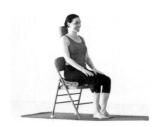

1   p158
Mountain Pose in a Chair

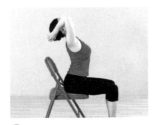

2   p158
Yoga Moves Your Eyes

3   p63
Backbend in a Chair

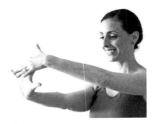

4   p80
Hand Press Wrist Release

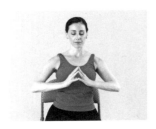

5   p85
Spider Hands Push-Ups

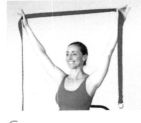

6   p76
Strap Happy

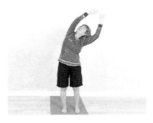

7   p103
Standing Side Bend

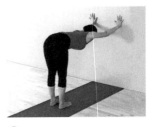

8   p305
Wall Dog Pose

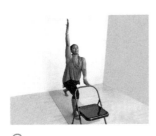

9   p166
Crescent Warrior Pose

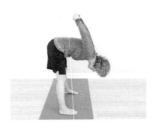

10   p320
Wide Angle Forward Fold Pose with fingers interlaced

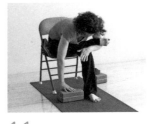

11   p130
#4 Pose in a Chair

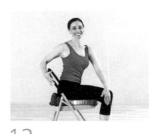

12   p271
Spinal Twist Pose in a Chair

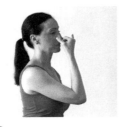

13   p32
Alternative Nostril Breath

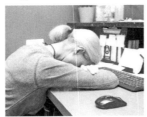

14   p248
Restorative Forward Fold Pose in a chair at desk

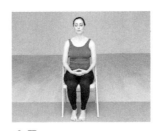

15   p238
Relaxation Pose in a Chair or Mindful Meditation (p22)

Ⓜ Restroom — "What Took You So Long in There?"

ENERGETIC QUALITIES: stretching, strengthening, balancing, refreshing

TIME ESTIMATE: 15 to 30 minutes

PROPS: restroom, countertops, wall, commode seat, dry body brush, massage oil or lotion

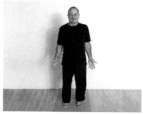

1   p220
Mountain Pose
(facing sink)

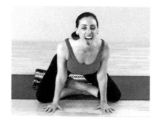

2   p35
Lion's Breath

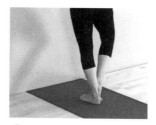

3   p293
Brush Teeth in Baby Bush Pose *Alternating opposite hands and feet*

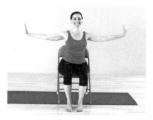

4   p84
Wrist Flexion

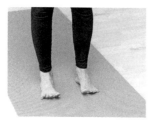

5   p118
Toe Lift — with hands on countertop

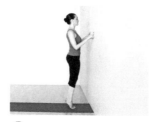

6   p119
Heel Lift with hands on countertop

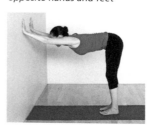

7   p305
Wall Dog Pose

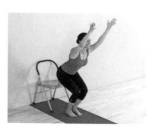

8   p150
Chair Pose ("Potty Pose") *Slowly and gently, lower and rise from commode*

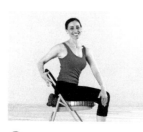

9   p271
Spinal Twist Pose on commode

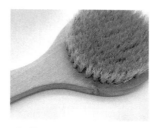

10
Exfoliate with dry body brush before shower

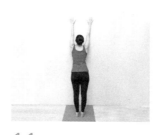

11   p76
Shower Pose

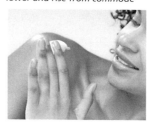

12
Follow bathing routine with moisturizing self-massage

Assess your restroom and ascertain safety to practice the sequence steps.

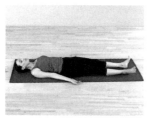

13   p238
Relaxation Pose

Ⓜ Against the Wall with a Chair

ENERGETIC QUALITIES: stretching, strengthening, invigorating, balancing

TIME ESTIMATE: 15 to 20 minutes

PROPS: yoga mat, chair, wall, blanket

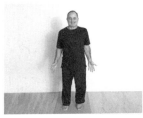

1   p220
Mountain Pose

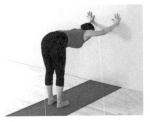

2   p305
Wall Dog Pose

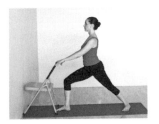

3   p166
Crescent Warrior Pose

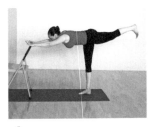

4   p314
Warrior 3 Pose

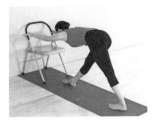

5   p236
Pyramid Pose

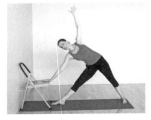

6   p300
Triangle Pose

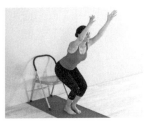

7   p150
Chair Pose

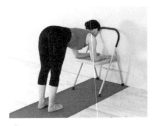

8   p168
Dolphin Dog Pose

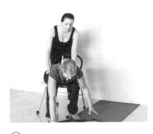

9   p341
Safe Landing: From a Chair to the Earth

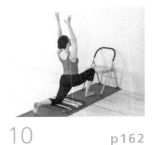

10   p162
Crescent Kneeling Lunge Pose

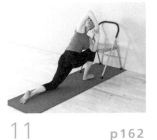

11   p162
Crescent Kneeling Lunge Pose with a twist

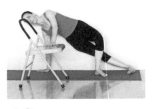

12   p265
Side Plank Pose with "Kickstand"

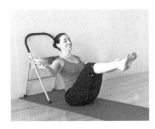

13   p133
Boat Pose

14   p215
Legs on the Chair Pose

Ⓜ *Anxiety Antidote*

ENERGETIC QUALITIES: calming, balancing, restorative

TIME ESTIMATE: 20 to 50 minutes

PROPS: yoga mat, blanket, blocks, soothing music, guided meditation or body scan

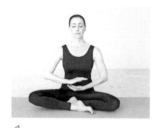

1   p175
Easy Pose, *Pala Mudra*
(p.335 optional)

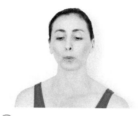

2   p175
Pursed Lip Breath (p29)

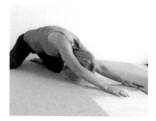

3   p153
Child's Pose Side Stretch

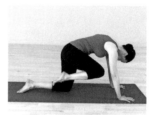

4   p283
Table Pose with Knee to Chest

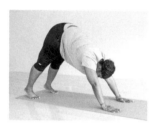

5   p170
Downward Facing Dog Pose

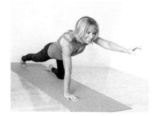

6   p268
Spinal Balance Pose

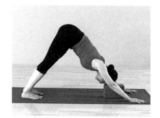

7   p170
Downward Facing Dog Pose with block at forehead

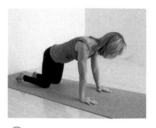

8   p280
Table Pose

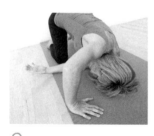

9   p291
Thread the Needle Pose

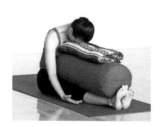

10   p247
Restorative Forward Fold Pose

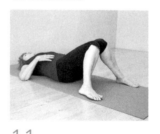

11   p32
Alternative Nostril Breath while in Constructive Rest Pose

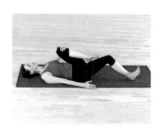

12   p108
Psoas Release on the Earth

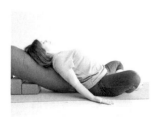

13   p245
Restorative Butterfly Pose

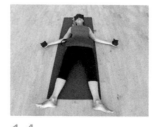

14   p238
Relaxation Pose with Yoga *Nidra* OR Body Scan *(refer to resources)*

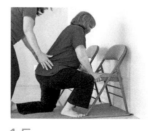

15   p343
Lift Off: From the Earth to a Chair or Standing

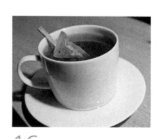

16
Enjoy a cup of soothing chamomile tea

Ⓜ *In the Kitchen Sequence Waiting for the Rice to Cook*

ENERGETIC QUALITIES: stretching, strengthening, balancing, invigorating

TIME ESTIMATE: 15 to 20 minutes

PROPS: kitchen, countertop, chair, wall

1   p69
Fingers Interlace
(standing in front of countertop)

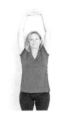

2   p119
Heel Lift

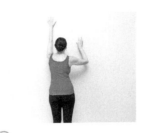

3   p77
Finger Steps

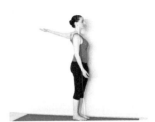

4   p73
Shoulder Opener at a Wall

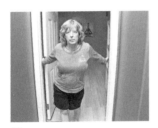

5   p79
Backbend between door frame

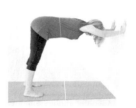

6   p305
Wall Dog Pose at countertop

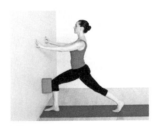

7   p166
Crescent Warrior Pose at Countertop

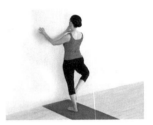

8   p293
Tree Pose

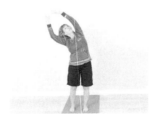

9   p150
Chair Pose against the wall

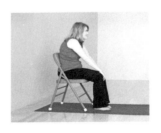

10   p103
Standing Side Bend

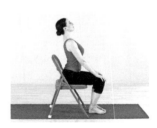

11   p148
Cat Pose in a Chair

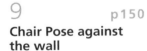

12   p148
Cow Pose in a Chair

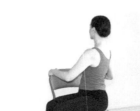

13   p130
#4 Pose in a chair

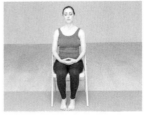
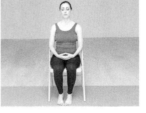

14   p271
Spinal Twist Pose in a Chair

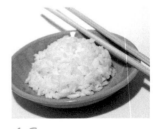

15   p238
Relaxation Pose in a Chair, *Dyhana Mudra* *(p.329, optional)*

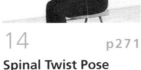

16
Enjoy the yummy rice!

Ⓜ *Took a Scenic Road Trip & Need a Break*

ENERGETIC QUALITIES: stretching, strengthening, refreshing, awakening

TIME ESTIMATE: 10 TO 15 minutes

PROPS: car, rest stop bench

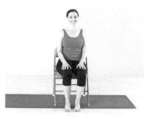

1   p222

Mountain Pose in a Chair

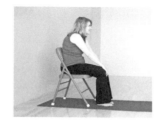

2   p148

Cat Pose in a Chair

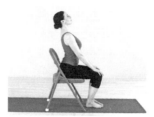

3   p148

Cow Pose in a Chair

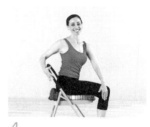

4   p271

Spinal Twist Pose in a Chair

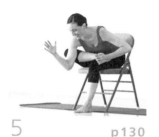

5   p130

#4 Pose in a Chair

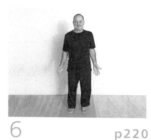

6   p220

Mountain Pose

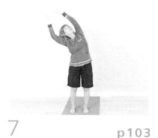

7   p103

Standing Side Bend Pose

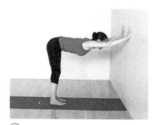

8   p305

Wall Dog Pose

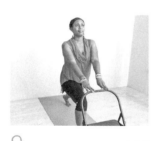

9   p166

Crescent Warrior Pose

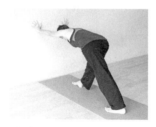

10   p236

Pyramid Pose

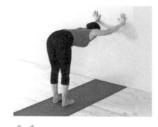

11   p305

Wall Dog Pose

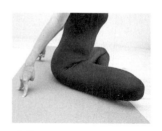

12   p222

Seated Meditation, *Bhu Mudra*
(p.327, optional)

For your journey, adjust your seat to support your lower back. You may place a pillow or roll behind your spine.

Before beginning the sequence, park in a safe place, and slide your seat back.

In poses 8-11, use the side of your car for a wall.

Ⓜ Yoga for Easing Transfers In and Out of Car Sequence

ENERGETIC QUALITIES: stretching, strengthening, balancing

TIME ESTIMATE: 15 to 20 minutes

PROPS: yoga mat, chair, block, yoga strap, blanket

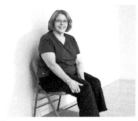

1   p123
Walking While Seated

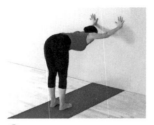

2   p305
Wall Dog Pose

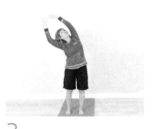

3   p103
Standing Side Bend Pose

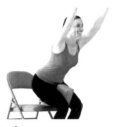

4   p99
Chair Pose Pelvic Floor Exercise

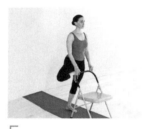

5   p293
Tree Pose

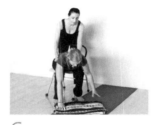

6   p341
Safe Landing: Transition to the Earth from a Chair

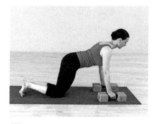

7   p280
Table Pose

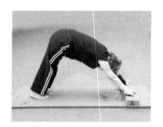

8   p170
Downward Facing Dog Pose

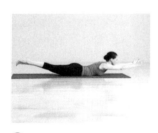

9   p218
Locust Pose

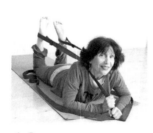

10   p288
Thigh Stretch Pose on the Earth

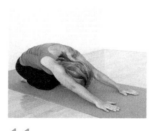

11   p153
Child's Pose

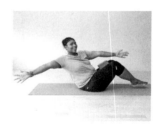

12   p133
Boat Pose with a twist

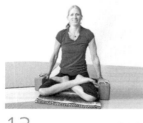

13   p258
Scale Pose

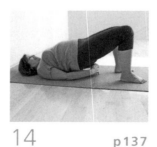

14   p137
Bridge Pose

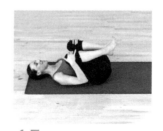

15   p106
Juicy Hips Spinal Massage

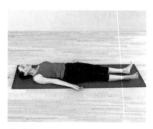

16   p238
Relaxation Pose

This sequence is designed to help prepare for the required actions to lift legs in and out of the car.

DEFINITIONS

Affirmation A positive statement to help bring a desired concept into your life. For example, "I am in harmony with nature."

Body scan A component of mindfulness, often guided while lying on the earth. Used to become aware of different parts of the body and their sensations, improve attention, and release stored tensions without trying to change anything.

Cactus arms A position of raised arms and hands with elbows bent ninety degrees and out to the side, like a goal post. Used when in standing, seated, or reclining positions.

Central nervous system (CNS) Comprises the brain and spinal cord and controls most functions of the body and mind. Processes information received from all parts of the body. One of the two major divisions of the nervous system.

Complete Yoga Breath A way to breathe using the diaphragm and abdominal muscles. A slow efficient breath characterized by inhalations through the nose, and exhalations through the nose or mouth. The belly, ribcage and up to the collarbone expand on an inhale, and the belly contracts on the exhale. Also known as the three-part breath or diaphragmatic breath.

Concave or lordotic Inward curvature of the neck and lower spine.

Convex or kyphotic Outward curvature of thoracic (upper back), and sacral (bottom) parts of the spine.

Crown Top of the head.

Curl Inward curve such as such as of the spine, arms, and fingers. Body action during a sit-up.

Dry body brush A skin exfoliation and detoxification technique used with a natural bristle brush to stimulate the circulatory and lymphatic systems. Often used before a warm shower or bath and followed by self-massage.

Diaphragmatic breath
See Complete Yoga Breath.

Earth In this book, refers to the location of the yoga mat. "On the earth" is synonymous with "on a yoga mat." Focus on the earth has a grounding effect. Touching the support of mother

Definitions

earth gives one a sense of steadiness and stability.

Energy Life force (*prana*). Energy can be physical or mental. The breath is directly connected to the quality of energy and the soul.

Energetically Refers to the quality of an isometric action. More subtly, refers to channeling energy through the physical body in a specific direction.

External rotation A rotation or turning away from the midline or center of the body.

Flex To bend or move a limb or joint by muscle contraction.

Floint To floint, point your foot, maintain the straightened ankle, and flex your toes toward you. (p117)

Foot drop or drop foot A general term for difficulty lifting the front part of the foot, stemming from weakness or paralysis of the muscles that lift the foot; often a sign of an underlying neurological, muscular or anatomical condition. The front of the foot may drag on the ground when walking.

Gait Description of how one walks.

Hamstrings These three muscles on the back of the thigh or upper leg combine with five tendons at the back of the knee.

Hatha yoga An ancient set or system of physical postures (*asanas*) and breathing practices that open energetic channels in the body and connect the mind, body, and spirit.

Heart center In this book, refers to the center of the chest (sternum), rather than the anatomical organ. A focus on the heart and loving-kindness to yourself and others is essential to healing.

Heart opener In this book, refers to yoga poses, often backbends, which open the heart area and lengthen the front of the upper torso, shoulders, and chest.

Hug-in To muscularly draw inward to the midline by contracting the skin and muscles to the bone.

Hyperextension Overextension of a joint with little to no muscle tone to support the joint, often in elbow or knee. Results in too much pressure on connective tissue, cartilage, ligaments, and tendons. Leads to injury with repetitive action.

Hyper-mobility A condition in which the joints move beyond normal range.

Internal rotation A rotation or turning toward the midline or center of the body.

Isometric Engaging muscles by channeling energy in a specific direction without moving joints and limbs. The muscles pull to the bone and contract, and resistance is applied against some force such as the earth, a prop, another body part, or a yoga buddy to a stretched muscle. Also, a type of stretch in which the muscles are contracted while stretching.

Karate chop A hand position made by pressing the pinky side of the hand into the earth, mat, or a wall. Term can also be applied to the foot.

Locked joint Fully extended joint, usually in elbows or knees, as opposed to a soft or bent joint. Placing weight on the joint may force it out of place. Joints that repetitively lock in full hyperextension can lead to injury.

Mantra A short word or phrase repeated during meditation for concentration; may be chanted, sung, or said to oneself without sound. Many who meditate choose a mantra or are assigned one by a teacher. An example is *Ohm* or *na-ma-ha* for their vibrational qualities.

Micro bend A slight, subtle bend in the knees or elbow joints. Also known as "soft" knees or elbows. Prevents locked joints, hyperextension, and wear and tear on joints.

Midline An imaginary center-line running through the body from the top of the head to the bottom of the feet.

Multiple Sclerosis (MS) A condition in which the immune system attacks the central nervous system (CNS), and communication to and from the brain and body is compromised. Damage to nerve fibers and the myelin sheath that protect the nerves leads to a myriad of symptoms. No two people with MS have the same experience. The symptoms include but are not limited to significant fatigue, muscle weakness, pain, numbness and tingling, spasticity, and challenges to balance, walking, vision, bladder, bowel, speech, swallowing, hearing, and sexual functioning.

Neuromuscular conditions A wide range of conditions that either affect the central nervous system (CNS) or peripheral nervous system (PNS) and/or the muscles regulated by that part of the nervous system; examples include ALS, Muscular Dystrophy, and Parkinson's disease.

Neurological The structure, functions, and diseases of the nervous system. Scientific study of the diagnosis and treatment of disorders of nerves and the nervous system.

Neutral pelvis Alignment of the pelvis in a neutral position; neither tilted forward nor backward. The front of the pelvis faces forward without a tilt to the right or left and at the midway point between anterior and posterior tilt (forward and backward) where the tailbone and sacrum lengthen down and the belly engages. Refer to Pelvic Tilt Pose (p. 224)

Neutral spine Natural curves present in the spine with the pelvis in neutral and optimal alignment: the neck spine curves inward (cervical); the mid-back between the shoulder blades curves slightly outward (thoracic) ; the lower back curves inward (lumbar); and the tailbone curves outward (pelvic). Refer to illustration (p.44).

Occiput The most prominently rounded part of the back of the skull.

Pelvic floor muscles Musculature at the bottom of the pelvic floor that is shaped like a hammock. The muscles connect the sitting bones, the pubic bone and the tailbone. Also referred to as diaphragmatic musculature.

Piriformis A flat band-like muscle deep in the buttocks near the top of the hip joint and sciatic nerve; hip rotator, helps turn the leg and foot outward.

Piriformis Syndrome Condition in which the piriformis muscle irritates or compresses the sciatic nerve; pain may be in the buttocks, and down the leg along the sciatic nerve.

Plug in Term to describe the action of moving a leg or arm bone into the center of the associated joint, hip or shoulder socket. To feel a plug-in with your arm and shoulder, first reach your right arm in front of you like you are grasping for something just beyond your reach. Then, with a straight arm, pull the arm bone back into the shoulder socket.

Prana Energy or life force, directly connected to the breath.

Definitions

Psoas Long muscle connecting the upper and lower halves of the body. It extends from the lower back, through your pelvis, and attaches to your upper inner thigh bones.

Restorative poses Poses that rejuvenate while relaxing and realigning the body. Props are often used to help align the body and to maximize the release of tension, stress, and fatigue.

Robot arms Arm position used in a reclining pose with elbows bent, upper arms and elbows pressing into the earth, and raised palms facing each other. Refer to Bridge Prep Pose (p.137).

Root To press down into the mat and earth like the roots of a tree.

Sanskrit Primary language of yoga; an ancient vibrational language that originated in what is now India.

Scalene muscles Found along the sides of the neck, these muscles begin at the first and second ribs, rise up the sides of the neck and attach to the base of the skull.

Sciatic pain Caused by compression or inflammation of the sciatic nerve in the lower spine, this pain can be felt in the lower back, hip and leg. See piriformis syndrome.

Self massage To anoint the body with warm oil such as sesame or coconut before, during, or after a bath or shower. Self-massage soothes, and invigorates the body and is known as *abhyanga* in Sanskrit.

Shlumpasana Posture resulting from slumping and rounding of the shoulders

Sickled ankle A misaligned or outwardly rolled ankle which can cause weakness; supination of the ankle.

Sitting bones Bones in the pelvis that create two bony protrusions on the underside of the buttocks; ischial tuberosities.

Soft joint A very slight bend in the joint to prevent locking the joint or hyperextension. Reduces strain on the joint by engaging muscles surrounding the joint.

Spider hands Shape of the hand formed with cupped hand and fingers pressing into the earth or wall, and looks like a spider.

Sternum Breastplate or flat vertical bone in chest area that connects the two sides of the rib cage in the front of the body, known as heart center.

Tailbone The base of the spine or coccyx. Lengthening the tailbone refers to a tucking or scooping action of this small bone.

Third eye Area between the eyebrows on forehead, considered area of inner wisdom.

Tripod of foot Three pressure points, consisting of the balls of foot just below the big toe and the little toe, and the center of the heel, form a tripod on the sole of the foot.

Yogi A male or female yoga practitioner.

Yogini A female yoga practitioner.

RESOURCES

BIBLIOGRAPHY

Fishman MD, Loren M.
and Eric L. Small. 2007.
*Yoga and Multiple Sclerosis:
A Journey to Health and Healing.*
New York, NY: Demos Medical
Publishing.

Hirschi, Gertrude. 2000.
Mudras, Yoga in Your Hands.
San Francisco, CA.: Red Wheel/
Weiser, LLC.

Iyengar, B.K.S. (1977)
Light on Yoga, NY: Random
House, Inc.

Kabat-Zinn, J.1990.
*Full Catastrophe Living, Using the
Wisdom of Your Body and Mind
to Face Stress, Pain, and Illness.*
New York: Delacourt.

Kabat-Zinn, Jon. 1994.
*Wherever You Go There You
Are: Mindfulness Meditation in
Everyday Life*, NY: Hyperion Books.

Keller, Doug. 2004 - 2014.
*Yoga As Therapy Fundamentals
Training Manuals.* Virginia:
DoYoga Productions.

Koch, Liz. 1997.
The Psoas Book, 2nd Edition.
Felton, CA: Guinea Pig
Publications.

Le Page, Joseph and Lilian. 2013.
*Mudras for Healing and
Transformation.* Sebastopol, CA:
Integrative Yoga Therapy.

Sanford, Matthew. 2006.
*Waking: A Memoir of Trauma and
Transcendence.* USA: Rodale Inc.

Stein, Amy, M.P.T. 2009.
*Heal Pelvic Pain: A Proven
Stretching, Strengthening, and
Nutrition Program for Relieving
Pain, Incontinence, IBS, and Other
Symptoms Without Surgery.*
New York, NY: McGraw-Hill.

Thich Naht Hanh. 1991.
*Peace is Every Step: The Path
of Mindfulness in Everyday Life.*
New York, NY: Bantam Books.

USEFUL RESOURCES AND ORGANIZATIONS

American Headache Society
americanheadachesociety.org

Center for Mindfulness
University of Massachusetts
umassmed.edu/cfm

Resources

Christopher and Dana Reeve
Foundation
christopherreeve.org

International Association
of Yoga Therapists
iayt.org

Multiple Sclerosis Association
of America
MSAA.com

Multiple Sclerosis Foundation
msfocus.org

National Fibromyalgia
Association
fmaware.org

National Multiple Sclerosis
Society
nmss.org

National Parkinson Foundation
parkinson.org

National Spinal Cord Injury
Association
spinalcord.org

Yoga Alliance
yogaalliance.org

Yoga Moves MS
yogamovesms.org

Yoga Props
yogaaccessories.com
huggermugger.com

SUGGESTED READINGS AND RECORDINGS

Bowling M.D., Ph.D. Alan.
2007.
Complimentary and Alternative Medicine and Multiple Sclerosis, 2nd Edition. New York, NY: Demos Medical Publishing.

Devi, Nischala Joy. 2000.
The Healing Path of Yoga, NY: Three Rivers Press.

Fishman MD, Loren, and Ellen Saltonstall. 2008.
Yoga for Arthritis, NY: W.W. Norton & Company.

Kabat Zinn, Jon,
Mindfulness Meditations for Pain Relief: Guided Practices for Reclaiming Your Body and Your Life (recording)

Lasater, Ph.D., P.T., Judith.
2011.
Relax and Renew: Restful Yoga for Stressful Times, CA: Rodmell Press

Meleo-Meyer MS, MA, Florence.
"living awake". *mindfulness practices for young adults* MA: Center for Mindfulness, University of Massachusetts Medical School (DVD).

O'Donnell Clarke, Karen. 2013.
Teaching Adaptive Yoga for MS Teacher Training Manual, Yoga Heals Us.

Sanford, Matthew. 2006.
Waking: A Memoir of Trauma and Transcendence, USA: Rodale Inc.

McCall M.D., Timothy. 2007.
Yoga as Medicine, The Yogic Prescription for Health and Healing, NY: Bantam Dell Publishing.

Saraswati, Swami Satyananda. 2009.
Yoga Nidra, India: Yoga Publications Trust.

Shah, Dr. Siddharth, Shah,
Yoga Nidra & Guided Meditation Self Hypnosis Techniques, Music for Deep Sleep (recording)

Stahl Ph.D., Bob and Elisha Goldstein, PH. 2010.
A Mindfulness-Based Stress Reduction Workbook, New Harbinger Publications, Inc., CA. (book and recording). (Note: includes body scan).

Stryker, Rod,
Relax Into Greatness (recording including yoga *nidra*, or "yogic sleep" for deep relaxation).

INDEX

Index

Index

ABOUT THE AUTHOR

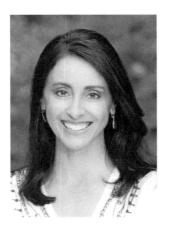

MINDY EISENBERG, MHSA, ERYT-500, is the founder of Yoga Moves MS, a non-profit 501(c)(3) organization. She has provided yoga therapy to individuals with Multiple Sclerosis, and neuromuscular conditions in southeastern Michigan for over 11 years. As a perpetual student, she seeks to learn from the best yoga and meditation instructors in the country. Her experience as a hospital administrator at the University of Michigan Medical Center contributes to her ability to bring the Yoga Moves philosophy of healing and the importance of the mind-body relationship to the health care arena. Mindy has a Bachelor of Science from Northwestern University and a Master of Health Services Administration from the University of Michigan.

NOTES

NOTES